The 10-Step Depression Relief Workbook

The 10-Step
Depression
Relief
Workbook

A COGNITIVE BEHAVIORAL
THERAPY APPROACH

Simon A. Rego, Psy.D., ABPP, ACT
and Sarah Fader

Foreword by Judith S. Beck, Ph.D.
President, Beck Institute for Cognitive Behavior Therapy

ALTHEA
PRESS

For the brilliant mentors who have guided me in my development as a cognitive behavioral psychologist. For the patients suffering from depression who have trusted in me (and CBT) to aid in their recovery. And for my amazing aunt Alice Rego, for the relentless courage and conviction she has demonstrated in battling this "silent killer" in our society.

—Simon A. Rego, Psy.D.

This book is dedicated to anyone out there who is seeking to help themselves. We hope these tools can help you lead a more fulfilling life.

—Sarah Fader

CONTENTS

FOREWORD

Every day, countless people struggle with depression—a very real illness. Fortunately, there is a highly effective treatment for this condition: Cognitive Behavior Therapy (CBT). Dr. Simon A. Rego—whose work I have admired for many years—and Ms. Sarah Fader have written an important workbook that distills the key ingredients of this evidence-based treatment.

CBT was developed by my father, Aaron T. Beck, MD, in the 1960s and 1970s. Since the first major study in 1977, researchers from all over the world have demonstrated just how effective CBT is for a wide range of psychiatric disorders, psychological problems, and medical conditions with psychological components. Leading mental health service agencies and policy makers have recommended CBT as a preferred treatment for depression.

Despite all of this, a challenge remains in delivering high-quality CBT to individuals who are depressed. Unfortunately, many clinicians don't use CBT or only use a few CBT techniques. That's part of the reason my dad and I established the Beck Institute for Cognitive Behavior Therapy in Philadelphia in 1994, where we train clinicians regionally, nationally, and internationally.

The lack of effective treatment points to the importance of *The 10-Step Depression Relief Workbook: A Cognitive Behavioral Therapy Approach*. This book details the core concepts and strategies from CBT. It also integrates mindfulness and acceptance approaches, as well as exercise and healthy eating. Readers will find helpful information on the nature and forms of depression, measures for assessing depression, tools to reduce their symptoms, and resources for additional help. Along the way, they will be provided with guidance on how to overcome various obstacles. They'll learn how to increase their motivation, identify their problems, create a plan of action, and attack procrastination. Interspersed with this information are stories and examples from the lives of actual patients, making the concepts easier to understand—and relate to.

This book will be useful both as a stand-alone resource and as a supplement to therapy or other treatments. It will also be useful for those who have recovered from depression, and for family members and loved ones, so they can learn about this highly effective treatment.

Whatever your reason for picking up this book, I encourage you to read it from start to finish and to practice every skill. If you do, you'll benefit from nearly a half-century of research that has established the strategies and techniques that individuals with depression need to implement to overcome their illness and remain well.

Judith S. Beck, Ph.D.
President, Beck Institute for Cognitive Behavior Therapy
Clinical Professor, University of Pennsylvania

INTRODUCTION

While it's perfectly normal for most people to experience mood fluctuations and short-lived episodes of sadness in response to life's stressors and challenges, *depression* is different. People who struggle with depression suffer greatly and function poorly at work and at school, in their social and family relationships, and in their home responsibilities. This is especially true when the depression is chronic (long-lasting) and is experienced at moderate or severe levels of intensity. In these cases, depression is no different in seriousness than any other medical condition. Yet, unfortunately, because we can't see physical evidence of it (like in the case of a broken bone), it often isn't viewed that way.

It's time to change our view of depression and see it as a real illness with serious—and potentially deadly—consequences. In fact, the World Health Organization (WHO) now lists depression as the leading cause of disability worldwide, and notes that it is a major contributor to the overall global burden of disease. In addition, at its worst, depression can lead to suicide. According to the WHO, close to 800,000 people die due to suicide every year (which equates to *one person every 40 seconds*), with many more people attempting suicide.

If you've picked up (or been handed) this book, odds are that you have been affected by depression, and you're not alone. Globally, it is estimated that more than *300 million* people suffer from depression. Here in the United States, depression is one of the most common mental disorders, each year affecting about 16.1 million adults aged 18 or older (6.7 percent of all U.S. adults), about 3 million adolescents (12.5 percent of the U.S. population aged 12 to 17), 2 percent of school-aged children, and 1 percent of preschoolers. Also troubling is the fact that depression appears to be increasing in each successive generation and starting at earlier ages. And the news is even worse for women, who experience depression at twice the rate of men—and this two-to-one ratio exists regardless of age, racial or ethnic background, or socioeconomic status. In people with depression, scientists have found changes in the way several different systems in the body function, all of which not only can have an impact on physical health but also can increase the risk of medical illnesses (e.g., heart attacks, diabetes, stroke, etc.).

While many different theories have been proposed to explain the causes of depression, most experts now agree that depression results from a complex interaction of social, psychological, and biological factors. For example, people who have gone through difficult life events—such as the loss of a job, the death of a loved one, or a traumatic experience—are more likely to develop depression. There are also interrelationships between depression and other medical conditions (e.g., cardiovascular disease can lead to depression, and vice versa). Making matters worse, depression can cause disability and dysfunction, which can worsen the person's life situation and, in turn, exacerbate the depression itself.

While many effective treatments have now been created to treat depression—for example, psychological treatments, such as cognitive behavioral therapy (CBT), as well as antidepressant medications, such as selective serotonin reuptake inhibitors—fewer than half of those affected in the world (and in many countries, less than 10 percent) are able to access these treatments. Barriers to effective treatment include a lack of trained health-care providers (which not only influences access to care but can also lead to inaccurate assessment and diagnosis), the social stigma associated with mental disorders, and cost of treatment (medications and therapy).

Given all of the preceding facts, the intent of this book is to try to overcome some of these barriers by providing a series of steps based on CBT, one of the leading evidence-based talk-therapy treatments for depression. We've also added some tips on how to stop procrastination, practice gratitude and mindfulness, and develop a healthy lifestyle. We believe that, if practiced together regularly, these steps can provide you with a set of skills that the research has found to help people with depression feel better—both in the moment and in the long term. These steps may be particularly helpful for milder forms of depression and in cases in which someone may be hesitant to use medications (e.g., with children and adolescents, or women planning to become pregnant).

There is an important part of the process to keep in mind, though: While we've laid out the steps detailed in this book in a simple manner, we are well aware that *simple does not mean easy*. It will take *motivation* and *commitment* on your part to try these steps. And it is perfectly normal for both motivation and commitment to waver at times—even in people who are not depressed. So, if you have a close supporter, it may benefit you to have them act as your coach (i.e., someone who can encourage and support you) as opposed to acting as your therapist (i.e., a trained professional who may prod into your personal life as well as give advice and teach skills) as you go through this book. After all, the research has shown that being accountable to another person often increases the likelihood of seeing a goal through to its completion.

In addition, if you want to maximize your chances of feeling better, you will also need to be *flexible* in both *how you think* and *what you're willing to do*. Getting better also requires *openness and honesty*—to consider that the way you've been thinking may not be accurate (especially when you're feeling depressed) and that the way you've been acting may not be serving your long-term goals—along with a *willingness* to try doing and thinking about things differently. After all, *if you keep doing what you've been doing, odds are you'll keep getting what you've been getting*.

Therefore, we challenge you to suspend any disbelief you may have and instead challenge yourself to read this book, practice the steps in a consistent manner, and see what happens. We've designed this book to be easy to read, with lots of practical examples (many from our own lives), along with worksheets, quotes, and examples to get you started and keep you going.

Remember: Depression is real. It is common. And it is serious. Fortunately, it is also highly treatable. We hope this book proves to be a helpful starting place.

Simon A. Rego, Psy.D., ABPP, ACT

Define Depression

More than just melancholy or sadness, major depressive disorder (commonly known as clinical depression) is a diagnosable psychiatric condition that affects each person differently. However, it's important and useful to know the most common signs and symptoms of depression; in fact, that's the first step in combating depression: defining what it means to be clinically depressed in the first place. Being mindful of the signs and symptoms of clinical depression can help you better understand what you're experiencing. It also gives you the ability to report your symptoms to your health-care professional so that they are better able to help you. If your therapist or doctor understands what you're feeling or experiencing when you're showing symptoms of depression, they will be better equipped to help you begin the healing process. Let's take a look.

Inside a Depressed Mind

When you hear the term *clinical depression*, you might think of a person who has some of the symptoms listed here—and perhaps that person is you. Do any of these nine symptoms sound or feel familiar?

1. Depressed mood most of the day

2. A pronounced decreased interest in or pleasure from all or almost all activities

3. Significant weight loss (when not dieting), weight gain, or decrease or increase in appetite

4. Trouble sleeping or sleeping too much

5. Difficulty paying attention and/or concentrating, often experienced as "brain fog" (i.e., trouble remembering things)

6. Recurrent thoughts of death and/or suicide

7. Excessive feelings of guilt and/or worthlessness

8. Feeling restless (e.g., leg-shaking, fidgeting, hand-wringing, pacing) or slowed down (e.g., slowed speech, slowed walking) in ways that are noticeable to others

9. Lack of energy and/or feelings of fatigue each day (e.g., difficulty performing small tasks such as showering or eating)

These are the symptoms of clinical depression as listed in the *Diagnostic and Statistical Manual of Mental Disorders: 5th Edition* (*DSM-5*), a comprehensive resource used by mental health professionals to diagnose mental disorders. Go back and place a check mark beside any symptom you are experiencing. If you have experienced five or more of these symptoms most of the day, nearly every day, for two weeks or more, it is likely you are living with clinical depression. If so, you know how physically and emotionally tiring it can be. So do I, Sarah; I've experienced it. Here's a snapshot of me dealing with depression before I got help:

> "I didn't want to leave my house because getting out of bed, showering, and going outside seemed like too much effort. I isolated myself from my friends, convinced that they found me burdensome, annoying, and tiresome

to be around. I found myself ruminating over negative thoughts and ideas of low self-worth. I had difficulty remembering things, and I found little comfort in activities I loved, such as writing, playing with my dog and cats, and singing. On top of that, my appetite was almost nonexistent, and I had to force myself to eat."

Does this sound familiar? Can you relate to my psychological state? I was coping with clinical depression. In this scenario, I had forgotten the things that previously gave me enjoyment in life. Due to my inability to take pleasure in things, I lacked the motivation to get going and engage in my normal everyday activities. I couldn't reach out to friends or a support system. This only made matters worse, because isolation can exacerbate the symptoms of depression.

When you are experiencing depression, try to remember that you are not alone. There are other people out there who are also challenged by an inability to perform even the smallest tasks due to depression. It can feel frustrating when, on some level, you truly do want to be with your friends, go out, and have a good time or engage in a hobby you once took pleasure in, but remember: You are experiencing a real medical disorder that is making it difficult for you to function . . . at the moment. And that's the thing: While depression may be something you are experiencing *in this moment, it can be overcome* when you take certain steps to feel better.

Now that I've opened up and shared with you a typical scenario of my own experience with depression, take a moment to reflect on the symptoms you've experienced and how depression has affected your life:

_____

_____

_____

_____

_____

_____

_____

_____

> WARNING! If you are experiencing persistent thoughts of death, suicide, self-harm, or other urgent mental health issues, put this book down and call 9-1-1 or go to your local hospital's emergency room. Having any of these symptoms means that your mental health needs to be addressed immediately. Remember, your life is important and life is worth living. You can also call the National Suicide Prevention Lifeline 24/7 for free and confidential support from a trained professional at 1-800-273-8255.

Depression in Your Body

Living with clinical depression is mentally challenging, but it also comes with a host of physical challenges. Let's more closely examine how depression may be affecting your body. Can you relate to any of these physical symptoms of depression, as listed in the *DSM-5*?

- Sleeping too little (insomnia) or sleeping excessively (hypersomnia)

- Low energy and/or fatigue

- Increased restlessness (shakiness, fidgeting, hand-wringing, pacing) or lethargy (slowed speech, slowed walking)

Have you experienced any of the physical symptoms of depression? In the space that follows, list the symptoms you've felt in your body and explore how you usually cope with them. Maybe these manifestations of depression have been too challenging to cope with; that's okay to admit. Take a candid look at your experiences with depression, and try not to judge yourself. Simply be honest.

_____

_____

_____

_____

_____

Who Is at Risk for Depression?

You might have heard that depression can result from chemical imbalances in the brain. While this is a widely held, yet controversial, belief, on its website, Harvard Medical School stresses that this disease is too complex to assign one particular cause. Depression can result from a variety of factors, including but not limited to genetics, serious illnesses, certain medications, difficulty with mood regulation, and stressful life events. For instance, people who experience a death in the family, a divorce, or a traumatic event (such as past physical, sexual, or emotional abuse) are often at risk of developing depression.

In many cases, trauma survivors are not only coping with depression but are also dealing with post-traumatic stress disorder (PTSD). Some symptoms of depression are similar to those of PTSD, including difficulty concentrating, feeling detached from others, trouble experiencing positive emotions, and trouble sleeping. Both depression and PTSD may also cause people to experience a decreased level of interest or pleasure in previously enjoyable activities as well as an increase of negative beliefs or expectations about themselves.

Sometimes there isn't an identifiable cause for depression. If that's the case for you, you know how frustrating this can feel. However, just because you don't know what caused you to be depressed doesn't make it any less real. Depression is as legitimate as any medical condition, and the reality is that sometimes we just don't know what causes it. The good news is that even if we don't know the cause, we do know that it's an extremely treatable condition.

The Depression Questionnaire

In the 1960s, Dr. Aaron T. Beck, a psychiatrist, pioneered the therapeutic treatment Cognitive Therapy (CT), also known as Cognitive Behavior Therapy (CBT). CBT aims to help people who are struggling with negative thoughts (e.g., "I am a total failure!") and maladaptive behaviors (e.g., sleeping too much, isolating from friends and family), which typically accompany clinical depression. CBT can help people struggling with these thoughts and behaviors by teaching them new skills in order to feel better. Understanding that depression has many different signs and symptoms that can range from mild to severe, Dr. Beck created the Beck Depression Inventory (BDI), which he designed to help people assess severity of the various symptoms of depression and identify the depth of their depression.

Since then, many other inventories and questionnaires for depression have been developed. Some of them (as with the one below) are aligned to the nine primary criteria for depression outlined in the *DSM-5*. This allows you to get a sense of the symptoms needed to be diagnosed with depression, how severely you may be experiencing them, and the total impact/severity of the depression, and it may help you determine whether or not to seek professional help.

The quiz below is the Patient Health Questionnaire (PHQ-9). Take this quiz now to get a better sense of your level of depression at the moment. Each question has four choices; write the number corresponding to the answer that suits you best on the line next to each question. You can take this test again in the future—either on a regular basis while reading this book, or at a minimum, after finishing the book and completing all the exercises, to see if the level of your depression has changed.

PATIENT HEALTH QUESTIONNAIRE (PHQ-9)

This depression quiz is self-scored. The scoring scale is at the end of this quiz.

Over the last two weeks, how often have you been bothered by any of the following problems?

1. Little interest or pleasure in doing things? _____

   0 Not at all
   1 Several days
   2 More than half the days
   3 Nearly every day

2. Feeling down, depressed, or hopeless? _____

    0 Not at all
    1 Several days
    2 More than half the days
    3 Nearly every day

3. Trouble falling or staying asleep, or sleeping too much? _____

    0 Not at all
    1 Several days
    2 More than half the days
    3 Nearly every day

4. Feeling tired or having little energy? _____

    0 Not at all
    1 Several days
    2 More than half the days
    3 Nearly every day

5. Poor appetite or overeating? _____

    0 Not at all
    1 Several days
    2 More than half the days
    3 Nearly every day

6. Feeling bad about yourself—or that you are a failure or have let yourself or your family down? _____

    0 Not at all
    1 Several days
    2 More than half the days
    3 Nearly every day

continued ▶

7. Trouble concentrating on things, such as reading the newspaper or watching television? _____

   0 Not at all
   1 Several days
   2 More than half the days
   3 Nearly every day

8. Moving or speaking so slowly that other people could have noticed? Or the opposite—being so fidgety or restless that you have been moving around a lot more than usual? _____

   0 Not at all
   1 Several days
   2 More than half the days
   3 Nearly every day

9. Thoughts that you would be better off dead, or of hurting yourself in some way? _____

   0 Not at all
   1 Several days
   2 More than half the days
   3 Nearly every day

Scoring: Total all the points that correspond to the statements you chose. Write this number in the space provided. (The highest total is 27 points and the lowest is 0 points.)

My score: _____ /27

How to Interpret Your Score on the PHQ-9:

0–4 points: no depression

4–9 points: mild depression

10–14 points: moderate depression

15–19 points: moderately severe depression

20–27 points: severe depression

If you scored question 9 with anything other than zero points, please seek immediate professional help. Scoring between 15 to 27 points generally warrants active treatment with psychotherapy, medication, or a combination of both. Does your score reflect your current mood? Why or why not? Did any of your answers to these questions surprise you? Why or why not? Explore your responses to these questions here:

_____

_____

_____

_____

_____

_____

_____

Identify Your Issues

Depression can manifest in many different ways and at varying levels of severity. It may also be accompanied by other conditions such as panic disorder, anxiety, ADHD, and substance abuse disorders, which are subtypes of depression; we'll look at those separately a little later in this chapter. In this section, let's look at conditions that people generally think of when they hear the term *depression*. These conditions include major depressive disorder (a.k.a. clinical depression), dysthymia (persistent depressive disorder), bipolar disorder, and postpartum depression. Regardless of the specific type of depression you're coping with, using this workbook can go a long way in helping you see the light at the end of the tunnel.

MAJOR DEPRESSIVE DISORDER (CLINICAL DEPRESSION)

A person who experiences major depressive disorder (also known as major depression or clinical depression and sometimes simply called depression) has a down mood and/or a decreased desire to engage in their daily tasks. To qualify as clinical depression, this change in mood and/or desire must persist for a minimum of two weeks and be accompanied by several other symptoms (mentioned on pages 2 through 4). The depressed or low mood and the resultant behavior differ markedly from how someone behaves when they're feeling their best.

People who are experiencing clinical depression must also report that the depression is causing problems in their work life, social interactions with friends, home responsibilities, and/or their academic career. Their significant shift in mood undoubtedly changes how they behave. For example, a student who has major depression may notice a dramatic drop in grades. This same individual might isolate from friends by declining social invitations.

PERSISTENT DEPRESSIVE DISORDER (DYSTHYMIA)

The symptoms of persistent depressive disorder, also called dysthymia, are similar to major depression but tend to linger on for months at a time. The symptoms generally are milder, though they affect the person over a period of years as opposed to the shorter periods associated with a major depressive episode. The level of intensity of the depressive symptoms experienced by someone with dysthymia can radically differ over the years; however, the hallmarks—low self-esteem, trouble with sleep, low energy or fatigue, appetite changes, poor concentration, and feelings of hopelessness—must not entirely go away for more than two months. Along with dysthymia, depressive episodes can co-occur, meaning that you can experience this low-grade feeling of depression along with a major depressive episode. In this particular case, it is commonly called double depression.

BIPOLAR DISORDER

Bipolar disorder (formerly known as manic depression) involves significant mood swings with accompanying behaviors, ranging from euphoric to completely hopeless. Bipolar literally means *two poles*; in other words, two opposite moods. The "up" mood is referred to as a manic (bipolar type I) or hypomanic (bipolar type II) episode, and the "low" mood is referred to as a depressive episode. People living with bipolar disorder go through intermittent periods when their moods are "normal" or "stabilized"—especially when in treatment with medications and therapy.

Contrary to popular belief, not everyone with bipolar disorder will have episodes of full-blown mania. People with bipolar type II experience hypomania (mild mania) during their "up" mood, which is not severe enough to impair their social or occupational functioning or to necessitate their hospitalization. In fact, it sometimes feels positive and they may experience periods of intense productivity. Unfortunately, the hypomanic light switch can turn off abruptly and transform into depression.

POSTPARTUM DEPRESSION

Postpartum depression is a surprisingly common form of depression, affecting one in nine women after childbirth. Those who experience postpartum depression have overwhelming feelings ranging from sadness to severe anxiety. They may feel thoroughly exhausted, physically and emotionally, and those factors make it challenging for them to care for themselves and their babies. Postpartum depression is not something a new mother brings on herself; it is as legitimate a mental health issue as any other form of depression and requires the same level of concern and attention as the other forms of depression.

Depression and Coexisting Conditions

It is possible that a person with depression is also experiencing one or more of the following coexisting conditions. Anxiety, for instance, may be a common condition that goes hand in hand with depression. What about you? Have you experienced any symptoms of these coexisting conditions? If not, do you think you might be challenged by any of them?

ANXIETY. Worrisome thoughts, feelings of nervousness, and uneasiness are all symptoms of anxiety. Feeling anxious from time to time is part of life, but when it dominates your thinking and activities on a daily basis, that's when it becomes an anxiety disorder. If you have an anxiety disorder, you may also experience feelings of extreme fear that seem to come on suddenly. This is commonly known as a panic attack or anxiety attack; we'll get to that in a moment. With regard to anxiety, Sarah's therapist once told her that depression and anxiety are two sides of a coin, and this made sense to her: After a period of depression, she found herself switching emotional gears to anxiety.

ATTENTION-DEFICIT HYPERACTIVITY DISORDER (ADHD). We're all familiar with that old stereotype of a person with ADHD: a child running around a classroom, unable to sit still and focus on the lesson. Today we know that ADHD also affects adolescents and adults. Symptoms of this disorder include inattention (difficulty focusing, poor school/work performance, poor time management) and hyperactivity and impulsivity (fidgetiness, excessive talking, interrupting others). Experiencing these symptoms can contribute to feelings of depression because other people may draw back when they are around these behaviors. This can lead to folks with ADHD feeling misunderstood, lonely, and even depressed.

(Note: Major depressive disorder occurs in a minority of individuals with ADHD. It's seen more commonly in the general population.)

PANIC DISORDER. This disorder is characterized by recurrent panic attacks, the sudden onset of intense fear or terror. The cause of a panic attack may be difficult to pinpoint. Symptoms include shortness of breath, sweating, shaking, and even feeling like death is imminent. If persistent panic disorder isn't addressed by a mental health professional, it can influence a person's quality of life. People with panic disorder sometimes isolate themselves because they feel misunderstood, worry about being judged, or fear doing something embarrassing if they have a panic attack in front of others. This isolation can contribute to feelings of depression. When Sarah experienced panic attacks, she did feel misunderstood and even weird, but there is a lot that can be done today to help you feel better if you're challenged by panic disorder. Please see your doctor or mental health professional for help; you don't have to live in fear that an attack will strike when you least expect it.

SEASONAL AFFECTIVE DISORDER (SAD). With the ironic, but appropriate, acronym SAD, seasonal affective disorder, like postpartum depression, nests within the depression diagnosis (that is, it is not classified as a unique mood disorder in the *DSM-5*). With SAD, episodes of depression have a seasonal pattern. For example, if you have SAD, you may feel wonderful in the spring and summer, but then experience a very low mood starting in the fall and continuing through the winter. On rare occasions, people with SAD experience depressive episodes in the summertime. You may have SAD if you experience the classic symptoms of depression exclusively in the winter months.

Do any of these coexisting conditions feel familiar to you? In the following space, reflect on your experiences, if any, with these coexisting conditions. If you suspect that you have an undiagnosed case of any of these issues, it's a good idea to discuss your symptoms with your doctor or mental health professional.

_____

_____

_____

_____

_____

_____

_____

_____

_____

_____

_____

_____

_____

Postpartum depression does not have a single cause; it can result from emotional and physical factors. After childbirth, a woman experiences a big drop in estrogen and progesterone as well as some thyroid hormones. These lower levels of hormones can affect the new mother's mood and energy levels, which can be a factor in postpartum depression. However, according to the *DSM-5*, approximately 50 percent of all postpartum depressive episodes begin before delivery, which is sometimes called *perinatal onset*. Don't discount these very real feelings, no matter where you are on your parental journey. Which type of depression do you most associate with? If you were to describe your depression to someone who is unfamiliar with what it feels like to be depressed, what would you say? Write about it here:

_____

_____

_____

_____

_____

_____

_____

_____

_____

_____

_____

_____

_____

_____

_____

_____

Review

This chapter covered what depression is in its various forms and how to identify the signs and symptoms. The first step to healing from depression is to demystify it, and we've begun to do that here. In step 2, we will examine a form of therapy that proactively treats depression, cognitive behavioral therapy (CBT), which was briefly mentioned earlier. CBT has helped many people break free of the oppressive chains of depression. In the meantime, think about what this chapter has illuminated for you, and write about it here:

_____

_____

_____

_____

_____

_____

Homework

Here are some concrete tasks for you to work on as you begin taking control of your depressive symptoms:

- Which symptoms of depression do you experience most frequently?

_____

_____

_____

_____

_____

- What provides you with a sense of relief from these symptoms?

_____

_____

_____

_____

_____

- Monitor your mood throughout the day—some people feel more down in the morning while others feel sadness at nighttime. When does depression hit you the hardest?

_____

_____

_____

_____

_____

- When you start to feel down, call a family member, friend, or someone else you know and trust. Reaching out to others allows us to get support and encouragement and feel more hopeful about the future. List the people you will call, along with their telephone numbers, here:

_____

_____

_____

_____

_____

STEP 2

Engage in the Therapeutic Process

When Sarah was pregnant with her son, she chose to stop taking her prescribed antidepressant under her doctor's supervision. She wanted to try a different form of treatment for her anxiety and depression, but she wanted to be sure to take care of her mental health during her pregnancy. She decided to try cognitive behavioral therapy (CBT) at a local clinic. CBT taught her an actionable skillset that helped her take control of her feelings of depression. As she used these tools, she found herself feeling better than she expected. Step 2 is all about engaging in this therapeutic process—so let's explore how you can use CBT to combat your depression.

The CBT Approach

Cognitive behavioral therapy, or simply cognitive therapy (CT), was developed in the 1960s and has since helped many people overcome all sorts of challenges. Before we step behind the scenes to learn a bit about the genesis of CBT, we want to assure you that this therapeutic approach has the potential to help relieve your symptoms of depression and anxiety the way it did for Sarah.

According to a 2015 article on ScienceDaily.com, an evidence review of alternatives to medication found that CBT can be as effective as antidepressants in treating depression. The goal of this therapeutic approach is to help you constructively cope with challenges that seem overwhelming. You're given tools to assist you in challenging negative thoughts. As you engage in this process, you will not only start to feel less depressed but will also start to notice a growing sense of confidence, mastery, and empowerment, which can help to prevent future episodes of depression.

A Brief Look Behind the Scenes

As we mentioned in the previous chapter, Dr. Aaron T. Beck developed CBT in the 1960s after conducting a series of experiments that failed to validate the prevailing (psychoanalytic) theory of depression at that time. As is the case with all good scientists, when his hypothesis didn't pan out, Dr. Beck developed a different theory. This led him to discover that integrated into the thinking of people with depression were distorted, negative thoughts and beliefs that were "automatic" in nature (i.e., often operating outside of their immediate awareness). As he delved deeper into the insidious role these thoughts played, he found that addressing them would be a crucial piece of a successful new therapeutic approach for depression, which he called cognitive therapy.

Beck also saw a distinct connection between *thoughts* and *feelings*. In fact, he coined the term *automatic thoughts* to illustrate how an emotionally charged thought could potentially enter a person's mind without warning. For example, you arrive at work late and are reprimanded. Your automatic thoughts might include "My boss thinks I'm an unreliable person" and "I can't do anything right." Feelings are then generated by these thoughts; in this case, perhaps shame and sadness.

Beck discovered that his patients were often unaware of these automatic thoughts, but with practice, they could learn to identify them and restructure them with the help of a therapist. Beck noted that if a person was constantly feeling emotionally dysregulated, their thoughts would likely be negative the majority of the time. Beck noticed that calling attention to these thoughts was essential to the patient's gaining insight into them. Once that self-awareness was achieved, the person could learn how to combat these thoughts and feelings and live a healthier life. Following this discovery, Beck began developing the CBT model.

Do you have automatic thoughts? If you can't identify any at the moment, don't worry. As you progress through this workbook, you will grow in self-awareness. For now, "listen" to yourself think, and if you can identify any negative thoughts, write them here:

_____

_____

_____

_____

_____

_____

Cognitive Distortions

Recognizing cognitive distortions, or errors in the way you are thinking, is an integral part of CBT. Are you aware of when your thoughts are distorted? The following are some common types of cognitive distortions with examples. If you relate to any of these examples, place a check mark beside them and take notes at the end.

☐ **FILTERING.** This involves focusing on negative aspects of a situation and filtering out positive ones. For example: You read the notes on a peer-reviewed class paper and focus on the one critical comment received rather than on the majority of comments, which were positive.

☐ **BLACK-AND-WHITE THINKING/ALL-OR-NOTHING THINKING.** With this type of thought, there's no middle ground. You are either on one side of the spectrum or the other. For example: You score 90 percent on a 10-question test. You see yourself as a complete failure even though you got 9 questions correct.

☐ **OVERGENERALIZATION.** This type of thought is generated by a single piece of evidence that is thought to be true for all other cases. When you overgeneralize, you tend to believe that when something goes wrong, everything is going to go wrong in a never-ending pattern. For example: You lose your job due to cutbacks and are convinced the same thing will happen at your next job and every job thereafter.

☑ **JUMPING TO CONCLUSIONS.** You jump to conclusions when you believe something is true without having any evidence to back it up. For example: You haven't heard from your friend, and assume that this friend is mad at you. Your friend hasn't expressed this, but you just "know" they're angry.

☑ **CATASTROPHIZING.** Here, you *predict* that something awful is going to happen. You expect to encounter the worst-case scenario. For example: You have a role in a community play and as you are about to go on stage, you think, "I'm going to forget all my lines."

☑ **PERSONALIZATION.** This is defined as seeing yourself as the cause of some negative external event, for which you were not primarily responsible. For example: You are on a date that does not go well and are convinced that it must have been your fault (as opposed to the two of you just being a bad match or the other person's shared responsibility in the experience).

- ☐ **CONTROL FALLACIES.** This involves believing that you are a victim of an outside force, such as the universe or fate. You may feel you are being punished for something, although you did "nothing wrong." For example: You lose an important document and believe that the universe or some other force is to blame because you are cursed by something outside your control.

- ☐ **FALLACY OF FAIRNESS.** In this cognitive distortion, you may feel like you are being unfairly discriminated against for some reason when things don't go the way you think they should according to your perception of fairness. For example: The train is delayed, so you are late for work. Your supervisor reprimands you, and this dampens your mood because you believe that it is unfair that you are being blamed for a late train.

- ☑ **BLAMING.** This type of thought holds other people accountable for your pain. For example: You have an argument with your partner and blame him or her for making you feel bad about yourself.

- ☒ **SHOULDS.** This is the thought that something or someone, including yourself, should be a certain way. Sarah's therapist once said, "Stop *shoulding* all over yourself." She laughed, but there is some truth to this expression; others call it "musterbation." When you think you *should* do or be something, it's often because you feel like you are doing something wrong. For example: You think you *should* do the shopping you've been putting off but watch TV instead, then you feel guilty about watching TV.

- ☐ **EMOTIONAL REASONING.** This distortion occurs when you feel a certain way and assume that the feeling is a fact. For example: You feel scared while flying and become convinced that *because* you're scared, it must mean there is a problem with the plane.

- ☑ **FALLACY OF CHANGE.** You believe that others will change if you want them to change bad enough. A person will change only if they want to change. For example: You are in relationship with a substance abuser, and you are convinced that if you want sobriety bad enough for them, they will become sober.

- ☐ **LABELING.** This is the use of unhelpful overstatements to describe yourself or someone else, like "I'm a loser" or "She's a bad person." For example: You refer to your coworker as "a complete idiot" because they made a mistake.

continued ▶

☐ **ALWAYS BEING RIGHT.** This is the thought that your view is the only correct one. Being wrong is not an option. Once upon a time, Sarah learned this expression: "Everyone is entitled to their opinion." Now, when Sarah is convinced that she is "right," she recognizes that there are other points of view besides hers. For example: You get into an argument with a group of friends who have a different opinion than you. You cannot fathom how they can all be so wrong.

At the beginning of this cognitive-distortion section, we asked you to place a check mark next to any of these dysfunctional thoughts you recognized. Did you relate to at least a few? In the space that follows, write about which of these thought processes you know you have a habit of engaging in and how you might be able to turn those thoughts around.

_____

_____

_____

_____

_____

_____

_____

_____

_____

CBT's Primary Principles

CBT relies on the foundational principle that your thoughts and feelings are inter-connected. The idea is to differentiate between your thoughts and feelings, and then begin to assess the validity of your thoughts in order to change how you feel and act. The graphic below is based on the cognitive model created by Dr. Beck to show the premise behind CBT. In any given situation, you may have an automatic thought followed by an emotional, behavioral, and/or physiological reaction. CBT aims to break down the situation into smaller pieces so that you'll experience the most rational reaction.

CBT IS FLUID

In CBT, you may be working on one area of your life and then find you need to switch to a different area to address a situation that has come up for you. With this flexible therapeutic process, you can easily flow from one life issue to the next and back again.

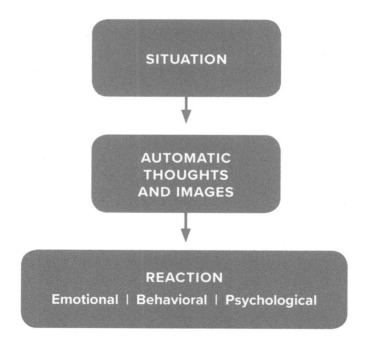

CBT WORKS BEST WITH TRUST

Trust is important in the therapeutic process. You'll need a certain level of faith that CBT works and that you will see real results when you engage in this form of therapy. Regardless of whom you open up to, be they a friend or a therapist (or even yourself), it is essential that you're able to trust that person. The work is more fulfilling if you feel comfortable enough to be vulnerable.

When you are working with a therapist (which we know isn't always possible for a variety of reasons), CBT is further enhanced by a trusting client-therapist relationship. A collaborative effort on behalf of the client and the clinician is very important. More than the other types of talk therapy, CBT relies on teamwork between you and the therapist. For a therapist to do their best work, it's necessary for you to make a conscious effort to work on yourself. Trust works both ways.

CBT EMPHASIZES CONCRETE GOALS

Unlike some other forms of therapy, CBT requires you to form clear and focused goals that you aim to achieve. For example, if your depression is keeping you from trying something new, such as a class, the goal of CBT will help you break this down into smaller steps, like looking for classes in your area, deciding which day might work best for you, and so on. Your goal is achieved when you are consistently attending the class. You may have one main goal for therapy or multiple goals you want to set. CBT can help you expand your horizons by either sequentially or simultaneously addressing several goals at the same time—but always taking things one step at a time.

CBT IS ROOTED IN THE PRESENT

CBT most often focuses on what is happening "right now" as opposed to digging in the past. It proposes that the factors that start a problem may be very different than the factors that maintain it; so, it gives you tools to help you focus on what you may be thinking and doing now that could be perpetuating your depression rather than requiring you to examine what occurred "back then" to cause it. This allows you to take action in the present and make changes that will not only help you feel better now but can also lead to a better future. This doesn't mean that taking a look at your past isn't helpful or never done; it's just not where CBT typically starts.

CBT PROVIDES SIMPLE TOOLS

Self-monitoring forms and thought records (see page 43) help you track your moods and activities and reflect on your style of thinking. These tools enable you to work on improving your mood whether or not you are actively in therapy. When you've learned and practiced these therapeutic processes, you'll also have an arsenal of tools to call on in the future to prevent slips and feel better in any given moment.

CBT IS SHORT-TERM, DIRECT, AND FOCUSED

Typically, in a therapeutic setting, CBT takes place over three to six months. A cognitive behavioral therapist will also welcome you back for some "booster sessions" or a "refresher course" if you want to revisit or brush up on the tools you've learned, review any challenging situations that have come up, and/or prepare for any upcoming stressors. When you choose this therapeutic process in a clinical setting, you will know what to expect. You and your therapist will collaborate on what you are working on and what your homework should be each week. This workbook complements that process, or you can start by using it as a stand-alone resource. The important thing to note, however, is that there is plenty of homework for you to do, as doing homework is critical when learning new skills!

Of the primary CBT principles discussed, which ones are most appealing to you? Why?

_____

_____

_____

Once you've learned some of the CBT tools, you'll be empowered to better face your daily challenges independently. However, as mentioned earlier, life is challenging at times, and depression can be sneaky and creep up on us. If you experience a setback, that's okay. You can always review what you did before and/or take a refresher course of CBT to help you get through a challenging time.

Other Types of Therapies

Since the 1960s, CBT has helped an enormous number of people find relief from the symptoms of their depression and other emotional challenges; it's definitely Sarah's go-to when she needs assistance through a challenging time. Others, however, may find that another therapy is what they need to truly feel better. Let's take a look at a few of them:

INTERPERSONAL PSYCHOTHERAPY (IPT). This is another excellent form of therapy that was first shown to be effective for people who struggle with depression, and it has since also been used with anxiety disorders and eating disorders. Like CBT, IPT focuses on what is happening in the present. And like CBT, IPT usually involves a limited number of sessions. IPT differs from CBT, however, in that it proposes that while depression may not be caused by interpersonal interactions, events that happen within a relationship can contribute to the onset or severity of a depressive episode. In addition, IPT notes that it's common for depression to have a negative impact on relationships. As a result, IPT addresses the interpersonal issues that seem most important to the start or continuation of depressive symptoms. These issues include: disputes with others, life changes or transitions that affect relationships, unresolved grief over the loss of a relationship, and general interpersonal deficits. In this form of therapy, the clinician helps the person build concrete social skills that they can use in their life to form lasting connections with others.

DIALECTICAL BEHAVIORAL THERAPY (DBT). Like CBT, DBT is a modified form of behavior therapy (BT), but while CBT focuses on challenging and changing negative thought patterns and behavior, DBT emphasizes balancing change with validation. DBT uses traditional cognitive behavioral techniques but also incorporates other skills (like mindfulness, acceptance, and tolerating distress) in order to help people accept uncomfortable thoughts, feelings, and behavioral urges. This form of therapy was originally created to teach people with borderline personality disorder (a diagnosable mental disorder characterized by unstable moods, behavior, self-image, and functioning) skills to cope with suicidal thinking and urges to engage in self-destructive behaviors, such as cutting. However, DBT is now also being used to treat other mental health disorders, such as bipolar disorder, eating disorders, addictions, anxiety disorders, and, yes, depression.

PSYCHODYNAMIC PSYCHOTHERAPY. Psychodynamic therapy focuses on a person's past experiences and how those experiences translate into the present. In this form of therapy, the therapist asks questions that help the patient find the answers within themselves. Psychodynamic therapy can feel freeing to the client, because they have the ability to discuss whatever is on their mind. It's the therapist's job to help focus these free-flowing thoughts to create insight and change.

BEHAVIORAL ACTIVATION (BA). Behavioral activation is a type of short-term therapy that typically lasts between 20 and 24 sessions. The therapist helps their client identify rewards, or "reinforcers," that encourage them to change their behavior. Behavioral activation teaches us that if we change what we are doing or not doing, we have the power to improve our overall mood. One technique that BA uses is breaking things down into smaller steps. For example, if you want to get out of bed, the first step would be to put your feet on the floor. We'll go into more detail about how BA helps people with depression in step 8.

MINDFULNESS-BASED COGNITIVE THERAPY (MBCT). MBCT is a type of CBT that focuses specifically on mindfulness. It has successfully treated episodes of chronic depression. This form of therapy combines the tools used in CBT with mindfulness exercises, such as meditation. Patients are taught to separate their thoughts from their moods. This form of therapy is based on the work in Jon Kabat-Zinn's Mindfulness-Based Stress Reduction program.

ACCEPTANCE AND COMMITMENT THERAPY (ACT). The goal of ACT is to modify the relationship people have with their thoughts and feelings that scare them. ACT helps people confront their fears and accept them for what they are. It uses mindfulness as well as acceptance to accomplish these goals. Patients learn to stop avoiding their fears and instead learn to understand them better. Clients have clear behavioral goals that they want to achieve. ACT is used as a treatment for many different mental health issues, including depression.

COGNITIVE BEHAVIORAL ANALYSIS SYSTEM OF PSYCHOTHERAPY (CBASP). CBASP combines elements of CBT and IPT as well as the psychodynamic model. In other words, it's an eclectic therapeutic model. The idea is that a person who persistently experiences depression repeatedly feels isolated from their environment and social settings. As a result, their relationships suffer. CBASP aims to help people form and maintain solid connections with other human beings. The therapist helps their client practice empathy and change the way they relate to others so that they can form longer-lasting friendships and romantic relationships. They are able to work on healing from past traumas associated with social dynamics. CBASP involves three main components: (1) situational analysis, where the client recognizes how their behavior affected another person and then changes their behavior with the help of their therapist; (2) interpersonal discrimination exercises, which compare traumatic relationship patterns with successful connections; and (3) behavioral skill training/rehearsal, where the client learns to be assertive with others in a healthy way.

Review

Engaging in the therapeutic process may seem daunting at first, but after reading and working in this chapter, you have a better idea of what sort of therapy is available to you. You even know that you can begin using CBT skills as you work through this book. Consider the possibility of working with a therapist, too, if that's feasible. We know that seeking help when you are depressed can feel overwhelming, but once you take that leap and find a professional who understands you, you'll be glad you did. Do you think therapy would be beneficial to you? Why or why not?

_____

_____

_____

_____

_____

When you begin working with CBT, you might feel like the process is slow-going—and you're right. It does take time to learn a new skill. Think of it like learning a new language or musical instrument—give it at least a few weeks of active practice. Hang in there; it will get easier, and you'll start to change and grow in ways you probably couldn't have imagined. In the meantime, think about what this chapter has illuminated for you, and write about it here:

_____

_____

_____

_____

_____

Homework

It's time to check in with yourself to see how you're feeling—and what you're thinking. Remember, whatever you are feeling is real, and you have a right to feel that way. But what you are feeling is connected to what you are thinking, and there may be cognitive distortions and/or problematic automatic thoughts influencing how you think and feel. Here are some to-dos to help you begin sorting this out, but don't worry if this seems too difficult right now. You'll have plenty of time to practice as you progress through this workbook:

- Practice noticing your automatic thoughts. This simply means consciously "listening" to your thoughts. Listen throughout the day in all types of situations and make note here of the ones you notice:

_____

_____

_____

_____

_____

- Can you identify specific times when your feelings and actions were influenced by cognitive distortions? In what situations or scenarios do those dysfunctional thoughts arise?

_____

_____

_____

_____

_____

_____

- What are the three most common distortions you use? Why do you think you use them?

_____

_____

_____

_____

_____

_____

Identify Your Problem Areas

CBT is goal-oriented, but before you can set realistic, achievable goals, it's necessary to identify which problem areas you'd like to change. That's what you'll do in step 3. This chapter covers some common themes people struggle with when they are depressed. We'll discuss coping with your "inner critic," dealing with major life challenges, reframing persistent negative thinking, and more. As you read, try to see which of these areas cause stressful and challenging emotions and behaviors for you. The area you resonate with most is probably the one you'll want to focus on when it's time to set goals.

To give you a sense of Sarah's own struggle with depression, here's an excerpt from her personal journal:

> "I've been sleeping a lot lately and I find it difficult to get to sleep at night. Either I'm sleeping too much or not enough. When I wake up in the morning, I don't want to get out of bed. I have racing thoughts that feel like a wave of anxiety, but they are too overwhelming to identify what they are. I try to push them to the back of my mind. I force myself to get out of bed, as hard as it is, and make breakfast. I don't want to shower because that feels too hard, but I make myself get into the shower. Everything feels 'wrong,' even though I am doing it anyway."

In this journal entry, Sarah is having symptoms of depression, but she is not sure what's causing them. The best thing to do would be pay attention to the thoughts to begin down the road of healing, but in this case, she pushed them away. She has learned a lot since then.

As we move through this workbook, we're going to keep prompting you to pay attention to your thoughts and continue to offer advice on how to do that. Our goal is to help you see them objectively for what they are (just thoughts), so that you can work through them and start feeling better. Yes, it's possible to feel better even in the midst of a depressive episode.

In step 2, you learned that the tools of CBT can help you find some relief from depression. But before you can start using those tools, you'll need to identify what your core issues are concerning your depression. It's important to do this so that you know what to target when you're feeling depressed. We're really going to explore this, but maybe you already have an idea of your core issue. If so, write it here:

_____

_____

_____

_____

_____

_____

What Are Your Core Issues?

People struggle in different areas when it comes to depression. There is a pronounced feeling of loneliness for some, while others find themselves overworking to avoid feeling down. It's important to dig deep to find out what triggers you into a depressive episode and/or what makes your depression worse. Let's take a look at some common factors.

EXTERNAL FACTORS

When you're feeling inexplicably down, it can be challenging to find the cause. When you're experiencing an episode of depression, a good place to start is to ask yourself, "What is happening in my life that is contributing to my depressed feelings?" Sometimes, depression is caused by an external factor that is influencing your mood.

Consider the situations that have contributed to your experience of depression, currently and in the past. When you analyze your thoughts and feelings, you may identify a common environment-related theme. Some examples of triggering situations include:

- Dissatisfaction at work, home, or school

- An upcoming presentation or review at work or school

- A traumatic experience

- A disagreement or problem with a loved one

- A major life change, such as a divorce, a child leaving home, or a death in the family

Note, however, that depression can also occur after seemingly "positive" life events, such as:

- The birth of a baby

- A promotion at work

- Graduation from school

- Returning from vacation

- The holidays or other special occasions

Take a moment to reflect on what environmental challenge you might be undergoing. Have you recently experienced a major change? Is anything happening in your life that could be affecting your current emotional state? Depression is affected by these outside influences, so try to recognize what those might be. What is happening in your life right now that could be triggering your depression? Write about it here:

_____

_____

_____

_____

_____

_____

INTERNAL FACTORS

There may be no specific triggering environmental issues, such as those discussed in the previous section, for your depression. As you probably know, there are times in our lives when everything seems perfectly fine, but we feel depressed anyway. Let's take a look.

Overactive Inner Critic

The concept of an inner critic falls into the category of automatic thoughts and dysfunctional thinking, which we discussed in step 2. The idea is that we each have an inner critic that comes out from time to time, judging what we say and do, and most often putting a negative spin on things. When your inner critic becomes overzealous and starts taking over your thought processes, the emotional effects can be devastating. An overactive inner critic can certainly contribute to the symptoms of depression.

Do you recognize when your inner critic is talking to you? The inner critic whispers things like "You're a bad person" or "You screwed up that project." The inner critic directly blames you when things go "wrong" in your life. Even when something goes well or a "positive" event happens, you can't fully enjoy it if that voice in your head is bent on making sure you see or think of only the negative aspects of yourself or your role in what occurred.

The first step to battling that inner critic is to recognize when it's talking. Try to become aware of what triggers those negative thoughts and what they are saying.

The second step is to acknowledge that these thoughts are separate or external from you. Yes, they are present in your mind, but they are *not* who you are.

The third step is to speak to your inner critic and tell it that you hear it, but you are not going to let it ruin your mood. Observe the thoughts as you would ocean waves or passing clouds. Mindfully watch them come in and out of your mind. Thank the critic for sharing its opinion, let it know you disagree, and ask it to move on.

These thoughts are important to pay attention to because when you know what they are, you can work on them on your own or in therapy. What does your inner critic say to you? Listen and write one or two of those messages here:

_____

_____

_____

_____

_____

Negative Thinking

Along the same lines of the inner critic, which tends to judge you harshly, negative thinking is a matter of judging other people and situations harshly. When our thoughts are focused on the negatives, we tend to see only the negative side of life. A big problem with negative thinking is that it becomes compounded; one negative thought leads to another.

When you notice that you are involved in a negative thought cycle, activate yourself by doing something like calling a friend, taking a walk, working on a craft project, playing with your pets, or doing some housework. The research shows that engaging in enjoyable and productive activities can get you out of that feedback loop of negativity and help improve your mood. For instance, if Sarah finds that she is caught in a negative thought cycle, she leaves wherever she is for a little while. For example, if she is at home, she gets up, puts her shoes on, and leaves the house.

We often don't realize how insidious negatively charged thoughts can be. Later, you'll learn how to use thought records to record your negative thoughts and put them to the reality test. For now, when you are caught in a negative thought cycle, what are some of the things you can do? Jot them down here:

_____

_____

_____

You have a right to feel your feelings, even if they are upsetting or disturbing. Remember, they are not who you are; they are just part of what you're experiencing—and more specifically, they are tied to your thoughts about what you're experiencing. It isn't what you feel but how you cope with those feelings that makes a difference in your life. You have a choice: You can succumb to your negative thoughts or you can learn to own your emotions and take back your power by using the tools you're learning and practicing in this workbook.

Rumination

Rumination is when a person obsesses over a thought or a problem repeatedly. When you're feeling depressed, you might ruminate on feeling "hopeless" or "not good enough." When you ruminate on these sorts of depressive thoughts, you tend to feel worse about yourself and perpetuate the pattern of feeling low or depressed.

What can you do when you're starting to ruminate?

- **Redirect your negative thought to a time when things worked out in your favor.** If you're ruminating about being dumped by your girlfriend, think about a great date you've had in the past with someone else. If you were able to have a good time on that date, there's someone out there for you to make more memories with.

- **Take a walk.** The thought you're ruminating on isn't going to go away. But you do have the power to take an action that will allow you to feel less uncomfortable. When you go outside, focus on what you see and hear. That will distract you from your nagging thought.

- **Call a friend.** Sometimes no matter how hard we try *not* to ruminate, it's difficult to stop. By calling a friend and sharing the thought with them, they might be able to do one of two things: (1) offer insight to your dilemma or (2) distract you with a funny story from their day.

Rumination is certainly a tricky monster to deal with, but you now have some tools to utilize to when you find yourself ruminating.

Unrealistic Expectations

Sometimes you may think that no matter how hard you work or how much effort you put into life, things don't work out in your favor. It could be because you have unrealistic expectations. These expectations may relate to your career, your love life, your health, or other aspects of life. For example, let's say you have been at your job for six months. You apply for a supervisory position, and you're convinced that you're going to get the job, even though Bob (who has been at the company for three years) also applied for the position. When Bob gets the promotion due to his seniority, you feel deflated. You just know you are better qualified, even though you haven't been with the company as long as he has.

We've all heard the expression "Life isn't fair," and it's the truth. Your suffering is *not* because you weren't capable of doing the job (or whatever else the situation might be). Sometimes things don't go our way because they are going someone else's way instead, and that's a part of life. Try to accept that while also focusing on the positive side and being grateful for it: You may not have gotten the supervisory position, but you work for a good company, and when another opportunity for a promotion comes up, you'll go for it.

Loneliness

People are social creatures; we crave interaction with others. If we don't get social stimulation, depression can set in. If we feel estranged from our family or if we can't find a social group we identify with, we may feel a strong sense of isolation. Not having a romantic partner and seeing others involved in relationships may also contribute to feelings of loneliness and isolation. It's also important to note that while we can become depressed if we feel isolated, we also tend to isolate when we are depressed. Once we begin to engage in this behavior, it may seem hard to break out of it, but there is hope.

If you are suffering from depression compounded with or caused by isolation, the solution is behavioral: try reaching out to someone. For example, you can set a goal to call someone each day. If calling someone seems too challenging, you can send a text. Texting is a totally valid way to reach out. Getting back into the mode of being social (or learning to be social) can take time when you're in a depressive episode. You're allowed to take it slowly. If you don't have friends or family members to reach out to, you can set a goal to find a meet-up group of people who share an interest with you. If you're looking for a romantic partner, a meet-up group could be a great way to find one.

We realize that reaching out isn't always easy to do. Sometimes you might just need to let someone close to you know that you're feeling depressed and ask them to be patient with you during this time. Who can you reach out to? What steps can you take to find a group of like-minded people? Write down some ideas here:

_____

_____

_____

_____

_____

_____

Seeing What You're Thinking

We've been prompting you throughout this workbook to share your thoughts in the spaces provided. Hopefully, you've been getting into the habit of becoming aware of what you are thinking and writing it down. It's especially important to record your negative thoughts so that you can see them in front of you (as opposed to trying to deal with them when they're in your head). When you see your thoughts on paper, it creates a little space for you to examine them more rationally and allows you to be in a better position to determine their validity. You can ask yourself, "Is this thought true?"

To determine whether it's true, you can look for evidence for and against the thought. For instance, is there any evidence proving thoughts like "Everyone hates me" or "I'm a terrible parent" or "Nothing works out in my favor" or "I'm going to fail that test"? We all have thoughts of self-doubt and that voice of our inner critic sometimes shouts at us, but we don't have to accept those thoughts as true.

Changing your negative thoughts into more realistic outlooks is challenging at first (especially when you're already depressed), but like any skill, it gets easier with practice. For now, all you need to do is write down your negative thoughts in the space provided below. You may also want to add a few loose-leaf pages to this workbook so that you can practice this exercise often. The more you do this, the more you will begin to see common themes and patterns. Start here:

_____

_____

_____

_____

_____

_____

_____

_____

_____

_____

_____

What's Left When I Let Go of My Thoughts?

Sarah once had a strange thought: "What do I have left if I let go of my thoughts?" She believed that her thoughts were who she was, but over time, she learned to see them as external to herself. It is common to be afraid to let go of the way you view things, even if the way you view things is toxic to your life.

Try letting go of your negative thoughts gently instead of trying to force them out. The research has shown that trying to suppress a thought or push it away only makes it more likely to be around. A classic example of this is called the "pink elephant" experiment: If we ask you in a moment to try your best *not* to think of a big pink elephant, with big pink ears and a big floppy pink trunk and a little curly pink tail, you'll discover fairly quickly that all you can think about is that pink elephant. Try it right now and see what happens. How did you do? So if trying to push out negative thoughts doesn't work, the goal instead is to stay relaxed (we know that's hard if you're anxious, but give it a shot), and let your thoughts do what they may. You're free to work on replacing negative thoughts with more realistic ones, but if you can learn to mindfully observe them and then let go of them without trying to control them, you may not even need to challenge them!

Replacing Negative Thoughts with More Realistic Ones

The expression "think positive" is easy to say, but it is not so easily done, especially if you are living with depression. In addition, sometimes thinking negative is the most accurate way to view a situation. The trick is to understand how depression taints the way we think and makes things appear more negative than they are, and to learn to catch and scrutinize what we are thinking in order to come up with the most realistic, balanced thoughts. The only way to get into the habit of this way of thinking is to work at it. Let's start now.

Take a look at some of the thoughts you wrote down in the previous section. Let's say one of them was "I'll never find someone to love." That thought isn't based in reality because you have no evidence to prove it. It's also cognitively distorted—you aren't a fortune-teller. A thought like that can be replaced with a more realistic one: "While I can't predict the future, I will certainly have a good shot at finding love when I'm ready to get out there and take a chance on meeting new potential love interests." That way of thinking decreases depression and gives you hope, and it's helpful because it leads to a productive action you can take to help your situation. Let's try another one: Let's say one of your negative thoughts is "The world is a cruel place." You can reframe that thought by saying, "While it's true that some aspects of life can seem cruel, there are also many positive things about the world."

Take a few negative thoughts from the previous section and try reframing them with more balanced and realistic thoughts here:

_____

_____

_____

_____

_____

_____

KEEPING THOUGHT RECORDS

Thought records are a key CBT tool for distinguishing between thoughts and feelings. Taking the previous two writing prompts a few steps further, thought records teach us in a structured way that we do not have to believe everything we think, especially when our feelings are negative (depressed, anxious, guilty, ashamed, angry, and so on). In fact, our feelings always influence how we think, so we can expect that with depression we will experience negative thinking—about ourselves, the world, and our future. When you use thought records, you are able to put your thoughts to the test and see what is valid and what isn't. When used properly, thought records help us change the way we think. With this tool, you'll begin to see a shift in your mood; you may even have a sense of immediate relief.

On the next page, you will find a thought record worksheet. Here's an example of how to use it:

Situation: Your friend Stacy canceled plans with you at the last minute.

Emotion: You feel sad, upset, and angry.

Negative automatic thought: "Stacy doesn't like me anymore."

Evidence that supports the thought: None.

Evidence that does not support the thought: Stacy and I always have fun together.

Alternative thought: Something important came up for Stacy.

Emotion: You feel disappointed but are more accepting of Stacy's need to cancel.

After you use the thought record, you should be able to view the interaction differently, like in the example. It's your turn now: Think about a life scenario where you felt a negative feeling and reflect on it with the help of this worksheet.

Thought Record Worksheet

SITUATION:

EMOTION:

NEGATIVE AUTOMATIC THOUGHT:	EVIDENCE THAT SUPPORTS THE THOUGHT:	EVIDENCE THAT DOES NOT SUPPORT THE THOUGHT:

ALTERNATIVE THOUGHTS:

EMOTION:

SITUATION:

EMOTION:

NEGATIVE AUTOMATIC THOUGHT:	EVIDENCE THAT SUPPORTS THE THOUGHT:	EVIDENCE THAT DOES NOT SUPPORT THE THOUGHT:

ALTERNATIVE THOUGHTS:

EMOTION:

Thought Record Worksheet

SITUATION:

EMOTION:

NEGATIVE AUTOMATIC THOUGHT:	EVIDENCE THAT SUPPORTS THE THOUGHT:	EVIDENCE THAT DOES NOT SUPPORT THE THOUGHT:

ALTERNATIVE THOUGHTS:

EMOTION:

SITUATION:

EMOTION:

NEGATIVE AUTOMATIC THOUGHT:	EVIDENCE THAT SUPPORTS THE THOUGHT:	EVIDENCE THAT DOES NOT SUPPORT THE THOUGHT:

ALTERNATIVE THOUGHTS:

EMOTION:

Review

In this chapter, we talked about identifying your core issues and coming up with a plan to manage them. Some of those issues include an overactive inner critic, loneliness, unrealistic expectations, negative thinking, and rumination. Once you know your challenges, you'll be able to set realistic goals for yourself. It can be difficult to see these issues clearly, because they may have been with you for the majority of your life. However, once you are able to recognize what's causing you to feel depressed, you'll be better equipped to develop a plan to strategically combat these issues. Remember, filling out a thought record worksheet when you start experiencing an automatic negative thought is an excellent part of any plan. What has this chapter illuminated for you? Write about it here:

_____

_____

_____

_____

_____

_____

Homework

Throughout the coming week, pay close attention to your negative thoughts to see if you can identify your problem areas. Are they related to your external environment, your inner world, or both? Consider questions like these:

- Do you feel unfulfilled in your work life?

- Have you recently gone through a major life change?

- Do you have a persistent inner critic?

- Are your expectations unrealistic?

- Is something else contributing to your depression other than these factors?

- What are the thoughts you are having?

- Is there a theme to your thoughts?

- Do your thoughts keep repeating?

Do what you can to really examine what's going on when you find yourself in a negative thought loop or feeling depressed. Jot down any insights you have during this weeklong examination here:

_____

_____

_____

_____

_____

_____

_____

Make a Plan

When you are depressed, making a plan might be the last thing you feel like doing, but take it from Sarah, someone who knows about this: Setting realistic, doable goals is key for getting through your depressive episode. Sarah knows firsthand that if she makes a list of goals she would like to achieve (goals that will improve her life) and begins taking steps to accomplish them, she will start feeling better. In this chapter, we'll help you figure out how to set realistic, achievable goals and how to respond to challenges as they arise so that you can keep moving forward.

The Goal Worksheet

This goal worksheet focuses on one particular area of life that you want to improve. We've laid out milestones within a certain timeframe for achieving your goal. You might be thinking that there's no point to this exercise or that it's not going to work. See how easy it is for automatic thoughts to creep into your head—even when you're trying to take productive steps to get better? So for now, let those thoughts be present, and fill out this worksheet anyway. You *can* do this. The first step is simply answering a set of six questions—let's get started!

1. What area of your life needs improvement? Your social life, your health, your fitness level, your career, or something else?

_____

_____

2. Reflect on your recent experiences in the area you identified. Choose a few of them and write about them here:

_____

_____

_____

_____

_____

_____

3. How much time do you want to dedicate to changing this area? For example, you decide to take a class to meet people with similar interests. Are you willing to spend at least an hour or two each week attending classes (maybe more if you invite someone out for coffee after class)? It's up to you to decide how much time you'll need to accomplish your long-term goal of making a change in the area you've chosen.

_____

_____

_____

_____

_____

_____

4. Set a short-term goal for yourself in this area. Using the example of the class, you could set a short-term goal of signing up for an upcoming class by the end of the week. To achieve that goal, you might devote 30 minutes a day for the next few days looking into your options: What topic or hobby, where (a school, community center, or some other place), when (what day or night), and so on.

_____

_____

_____

_____

_____

_____

continued ▶

5. Create a plan to achieve your goal of improving this area of your life. Keep in mind that taking a class might be just one step to achieving your overall plan. Part of your plan could include an accountability partner—someone who has agreed to hold you responsible for completing your milestones. For example, when you sign up for the class, you would report your accomplishment to your partner, or your partner might check in with you to see if you've accomplished what you set out to do. Even better—have them take the class with you!

_____

_____

_____

_____

_____

6. It's action time! Set your plan into motion and keep track of your progress. You might have to make adjustments as time goes by. For example, maybe that class doesn't start for a month, but you want to start making improvements now. You can brainstorm other ideas for moving toward your goal. And guess what? That's perfectly okay. Life is a process, and so is setting and achieving goals.

_____

_____

_____

_____

_____

_____

Overcoming Common Obstacles to Achieving Your Goals

When you set a goal, regardless of how big or small, you will most certainly encounter an obstacle or two (or more) along the way. You can either give up or figure a way around that obstacle in your path. We know you'll choose the second option because you're using this workbook for a reason. So let's take a look at some of the things that may block your way—these are things you can't necessarily prevent, but you can prepare for them and change how you approach them.

REFRAME THE WORD *OBSTACLE* TO *CHALLENGE*

When Sarah is afraid to risk something new to achieve a goal, she calls upon a quote from Frank Herbert's novel, *Dune*: "Fear is the mind killer." Fear can stop you from moving forward, but only if you let it. When you're feeling depressed, the word *obstacle* and the thought of encountering an obstacle can be perceived as a threat. However, if you reframe this thought and look at threats and obstacles as challenges, you're halfway to a solution. When you are faced with a challenge, you have an opportunity to use your creative thinking skills.

> *"Obstacles are those frightful things you see when you take your eyes off your goal."*
>
> —Henry Ford

Actively solving your problems creates a chance to grow. All you need to do is access your mental toolbox. A challenge doesn't mean you're blocked from succeeding; it means you can try multiple methods and see which one works the best. Here's an example: You feel like a failure because you're having trouble getting to your fitness class five days a week due to your demanding work schedule. So, you decide to attend the class three days a week and ride your bike throughout your neighborhood two days a week. The fitness plan wasn't working due to the challenge of having a full-time job. But you found a way around that by creating a more realistic schedule.

Nobody is dictating how you should live your life, so flexibly adjust your plans so they work better for you. You are not destined to fail, and you don't have to give into that idea. If you focus on failing, you're more likely to feel guilt and shame. That is going to be a further barrier to achieving your goals. Remember, the fear of failing is bound to come up. It's what you do with that fear that matters.

AVOID CATASTROPHIZING

When we discussed cognitive distortions in step 2, we talked about catastrophizing. It is the distorted belief that something is (or will be) way worse than it is. It's important to look out for catastrophizing when you are setting and pursuing your goals. You want to train your brain to catch this distortion if it appears, and then focus your attention on the present as opposed to fixating on the future. You have a goal in mind, but to reach it, you'll increase your chances of success if you remain in the present, taking things one step at a time.

There are two common forms of catastrophizing to be aware of:

1. **Perceiving a disaster based on one situation.** For example: You have one fight with your romantic partner, and you believe you're going to break up. One fight does not a breakup make. But if you're in the mode of catastrophizing, you honestly believe that this is going to be the outcome of that fight.

2. **Worrying about the future (or what's to come) and seeing a negative outcome.** For example: You imagine the future will be filled with things that are awful and bound to go awry. It feels like an alternate universe where you are a distorted, dislikable version of yourself. After you've "seen" this outcome, you imagine and develop a framework around this new reality. You are convinced that this dark world will come to fruition.

We're fairly certain that, if you had a choice, you wouldn't *want* to think the worst-case scenario will occur. However, you may not even *realize* you are catastrophizing. If you want to stop thinking that things will go wrong, pay attention to when you're having those thoughts. Once you're able to see the pattern of distorted thinking, you'll be in the best position to stop it. If you want a clue as to when you might be catastrophizing, look at your emotions—chances are you'll be feeling anxious.

Begin taking note of when you start having catastrophic thoughts about the future. Write them in the space that follows when they come up (or on whatever paper is handy—or even in a notes app—if you don't have this workbook with you).

First, write down what happened in the situation, making sure to focus on the facts as if you were describing a crime scene to a police officer. After you've recorded the objective facts, move on to your subjective thoughts and feelings about the situation.

_____

_____

_____

_____

_____

_____

_____

Read aloud what you wrote to make the negative thinking clearer and more pronounced. If you do this each time worries about the future start overwhelming you, in a relatively short period of time, you'll notice that catastrophizing is often linked to certain areas of your life. Understanding that this myopic thinking occurs in patterns makes it much easier to develop a plan to change it.

In general, what leads you to catastrophize?

_____

_____

_____

What specific situations often lead you to think the worst?

_____

_____

_____

In these situations, what are some common negative thoughts you have?

_____

_____

_____

Think of a specific situation you've recently experienced. If you were in that situation now, how might you reframe your thought process and stop catastrophizing?

_____

_____

_____

SMART GOALS

What are SMART goals? They are *Specific, Measurable, Attainable, Rewarding,* and *Time-limited.* When you set a goal, you want to make sure that it's precise. You'll want to make sure that the goal has a way of being tracked or measured. Additionally, your goal should be something that feels rewarding to you, and it needs to be achieved by a certain time. Sarah knows that she doesn't accomplish anything without setting a deadline, so she believes that setting an end date for your goal will help you, too. Let's get into how to achieve your goals now.

One reason why a goal isn't achieved is because it's too general. Saying, "I want to lose weight" is too broad. Instead, define how many pounds you want to lose and in what period of time. It's good to have a starting point, but once you have that marker, it's time to get specific and define your plan to the letter. Another thing to consider is, "Do I need to work with a professional to achieve this goal?" Weight loss is a great example of this. You should consult a medical professional before you start embarking on changing your diet or developing a fitness plan.

Let's say you want to curb your impulsivity. Maybe you have a problem with calling or texting people at inappropriate hours. You may want to speak to a therapist or mental health professional since this is a behavioral issue. You run into an obstacle when you say, "I am going to stop doing *X.*" It's difficult to just "stop" doing something. It's more realistic to do something to decrease an unhealthy behavior

A Common Roadblock in Goal-Setting

Setting a goal that you *don't* really want will stop you in your tracks every time, so be sure you are setting goals that resonate with you. Try this now: Think of a specific goal you *think* you would like to set, and respond to the following three questions:

1. Why do you want to achieve this particular goal?

_____

_____

_____

2. How will attaining this goal help you in the short term?

_____

_____

_____

3. How will it affect your life for the better in the long term?

_____

_____

_____

When you're setting goals, the most important thing to remember is that they are for *you*—not for your family member, friend, or partner. You're working toward your goals to improve your quality of life, so before you set any goal, sit with it for a moment, get real, look inside, and ask yourself those three questions.

and/or substitute it with a healthier one. So, you can say, "After 9:00 P.M., if I want to call or text someone, I will write them an e-mail instead. This way, they can read it at their leisure."

SET SMALLER GOALS

Think about where you want to end up and then work backward. There are times when your goal is so large that it may seem unattainable. When you think about a realistic goal, it will feel like you could possibly get to where you're going; but if you're aiming too high, you're more likely to feel paralyzed and think there's no point in moving forward.

Don't fall into that kind of negative thinking. You can do it, whatever "it" is. Maybe you want to run a 5K, but you've never run for more than 15 minutes at a time. You can start with an app like Couch to 5K (c25k.com/mobile), which will help you incrementally do what you need to do to become a runner.

Think about it like this: Imagine you are looking at a mountain. When you see the peak, it seems so far away. You can't imagine how you'll get to the top. You don't need to worry about that right now. Focus on one step at a time, and before you know it, you'll have mounted the peak. Don't say, "In no time," because it does take time to get to the top—just like it takes time to achieve your ultimate goal. Keep at it, and you'll be able to finish.

JUST DO IT . . . REALLY

A good friend once told Sarah, "I'm focusing on what I'm *doing*, not on how I'm *feeling*." And she took that simple statement to heart. When she is having trouble pushing through a depressive episode, she thinks of the well-known Nike slogan: *Just do it*. Negative thoughts will come and go, but Sarah has the power to choose to keep going, even if they are running alongside her.

This is especially relevant to setting and achieving goals. Yes, you're feeling depressed, but that doesn't mean you can't still keep going and take action. You may not feel better immediately, but over time, your mood will shift if you pro-actively work toward your goals.

Simon shares with us a great analogy developed by Steven Hayes, who developed acceptance and commitment therapy (ACT). It's the "passengers on the bus" analogy. Your life is like riding on a bus. You're the driver and on the road you pick up passengers. Some passengers don't have an effect on you, while others come into play when you've developed a new romantic relationship or made a career change. Some passengers hold more significance than others. The key to achieving your goals is to notice when there are difficult or challenging passengers on your life-bus and find a way to deal with them. These are both the people who enter your life and the internal passengers you are coping with. When thinking about goal achievement, it's important to pay attention to what beliefs these passengers (both internal and external) are having on the road of your life. Integrate the positive influences and ask the negative ones to get off at the next stop.

In life, we are not guaranteed an outcome. The best we can do is work hard, and the rest is in front of us. You do have control over your thoughts and actions, and that is a big part of achieving success. Here are two ways to help you "just do it":

"Individuals who procrastinate frequently confuse motivation and action. You foolishly wait until you feel in the mood to do something. Since you don't feel like doing it, you automatically put it off.

"Your error is your belief that motivation comes first, and then leads to activation and success.

"But it is usually the other way around; action must come first, and the motivation comes later on."

—David Burns

1. **Have hope.** Depression tries to convince you that there is no hope, so you should stop trying. This is a lie, and you don't need to believe this, but you *do* need to keep going. As you go toward your goal, you may continue to feel like there is no point, or dwell on failures, but remind yourself that there is a light at the end of the tunnel, even if you can't see it. Don't punish yourself for negative thoughts. Your mind isn't you. Allow your thoughts to enter your brain, acknowledge them (either mentally or by writing them down), and continue working on a step toward your goal, holding on to the hope that you will reach the finish line.

2. **Remind yourself of your own strength.** When you're feeling down, it's difficult to remember what it's like to feel good about yourself. One way to start feeling better is to remind yourself of a time in the past that was challenging and how you got through it. Making life changes is hard, but it's easier when you believe that if you've done it before you can do it again. You got through that time because you believed in yourself. Ultimately, it's your dedication and passion to change that will help you achieve your goals. You have the power to help yourself feel better.

Goal Progress Worksheet

Staying on track is key to achieving your goals. A week after you set your goal, it's time to check in. This worksheet helps you continue working toward your goal even if you're feeling a bit burned-out. When the weekly check-in rolls around, remember the earlier advice to "just do it."

Try not to judge yourself as you fill out this worksheet. There are many milestones along the way to achieving your goals. You may not be where you want to be, but you're getting there. There's no wrong or right here. The only person you're reporting to is *yourself*. As you answer the following 10 questions, be honest with yourself concerning your strengths and where you need to make some adjustments. We believe in you! Now let's get cracking.

1. What are your feelings toward the area of your life in which you set a goal to improve? Why do you think you feel that way?

_____

_____

_____

_____

_____

2. What was your most recent feeling of accomplishment with regard to this goal?

_____

_____

_____

_____

_____

3. What was your most recent experience of feeling challenged? What did you do when you encountered that challenge?

_____

_____

_____

_____

_____

4. How much time are you devoting to making a change in this area of your life?

_____

_____

_____

_____

_____

5. What are your short-term goals with regard to this change? Are you meeting those goals?

_____

_____

_____

_____

_____

continued ▶

6. Do you need to modify or change anything in your plan to help you achieve your goal? If so, what modifications do you need to make?

_____

_____

_____

_____

_____

7. Have you completed any milestones? What are they?

_____

_____

_____

_____

_____

8. What is a change you've made that you're proud of? Why?

_____

_____

_____

_____

_____

9. What is something that needs to be improved in your plan?

_____

_____

_____

_____

_____

10. What are your next steps toward your goal? Create a to-do list:

_____

_____

_____

_____

_____

_____

_____

_____

_____

_____

_____

_____

continued ▶

TRACKING YOUR GOALS

Review your goal worksheet alongside your completed goal-progress worksheet to see how far you've come. Were there any surprises? When you first filled out your goal worksheet, it may have felt overwhelming, but now that you can see some progress, maybe you're feeling more in control and hopeful about reaching your goals. Only you know how you're feeling. In the following space, write about what setting these goals has done for you so far and how you feel about them.

_____

_____

_____

_____

_____

_____

Review

Setting and achieving goals is all part of making a plan, the fourth step in this ten-step process toward feeling better. To achieve your goals, you need to make them realistic and doable. Remember what we covered in this chapter:

- Start small.

- Be specific.

- Set realistic goals in a reasonable time frame.

- Be patient with yourself.

- Avoid catastrophizing and negative thinking.

- Just do it.

- Use the worksheets to set goals and track your progress.

These points are crucial to help you stay on track so you can get to where you're going. It can be challenging to reach your goals if you're constantly thinking about the end goal. Try not to worry about the end goal, and stay in the moment. It might be a rocky path, but you have the tools within you to meet those challenges via your ability to problem solve. You will get there, but it will take time and dedication to reach your destination. In the meantime, think about what this chapter has illuminated for you, and write about it here:

_____

_____

_____

_____

_____

_____

_____

Homework

If you haven't already done so, now is the time to create a goal worksheet. Choose a specific goal and fill out the goal worksheet outlined on pages 48 to 50. If you need more paper, just get some loose-leaf pages so you can fold them into this workbook. Remember to be realistic about what you can achieve in a finite amount of time.

After creating your goal worksheet, set a reminder to check in at the end of each day. Fill out the goal-progress worksheet. This helps you monitor your progress and creates a sense of structure around your goal.

This is optional, but if you think it will help, choose an accountability partner (someone you trust and with whom you feel comfortable sharing your experiences). This is a person you can check in with when you're working on a goal. When you say you're going to do X by a certain date, you can report to that person that you did it. Having someone cheer for you is a wonderful reward for all your hard work. They may even want to join you on your goal. If you've chosen an accountability partner, write that person's name and contact information here, as well as the dates on which you need to check in with that person:

_____

_____

_____

_____

_____

_____

_____

Understand and Identify Negative Thought Patterns

We discussed negative thought patterns earlier in this workbook, but with step 5, we're really going to get into the nitty-gritty of it all and more deeply explore what negative thoughts are, how to identify them, and how to work with them to feel better.

This isn't about getting rid of negative thoughts completely, but more about how we cope with them. For example, Sarah has a negative core belief that everything she says or does is wrong. It's been with her as far back as she can remember. She is always working on reframing it, but she knows the process takes time. During a recent conflict with a friend, her negative core belief was triggered and she began to think that she was a bad friend, which then triggered feelings of shame and sadness. She began to cry and felt as if she was spiraling out of control. Then she remembered to use the tools we are teaching you about in this workbook. She shares this as a great example of how negative thoughts can influence us on a deep level and how important it is to use CBT skills in the moment. Let's keep going.

Where Do Negative Thoughts Come From?

Whether you're depressed or not, it's perfectly normal to have uncomfortable thoughts without being able to identify where they came from or why you can't get rid of them. In many cases, negative core beliefs, which trigger negative thoughts and uncomfortable feelings, can be traced back to childhood—perhaps you experienced ongoing trauma, a single traumatic incident, abuse, other impactful life experience, or even misunderstandings of what was happening around you.

Is it possible that an incident or experiences during your childhood may have contributed to the negative thoughts and feelings you have today? For some insight, respond to the following four questions:

1. Did any of your childhood experiences convince you that there was something wrong with you? If so, what did you think was wrong?

_____

_____

_____

_____

_____

2. Are there particular situations you associate with the negative thoughts and feelings you have about yourself? Do these scenarios affect how you view yourself?

_____

_____

_____

_____

_____

3. Is there one person you associate with these incidents? In what way has this person influenced how you feel about yourself?

_____

_____

_____

_____

_____

4. What words are you using to describe yourself based on this memory or trauma?

_____

_____

_____

_____

_____

Two Exercises for Sorting Through Negative Memories

You don't need to know the exact origins of your negative thoughts in order to feel better, so if you didn't gain any insight into your childhood from the writing prompts, don't worry. You can still move forward. However, if you did identify negative or traumatic experiences, here are additional exercises you may want to try:

- Journal about your experiences in a constructive way by visualizing yourself at your current age in a situation that you feel contributed to your negative core belief. Knowing what you know now, how would you have handled the situation differently? Spend a few minutes writing about some alternative reactions you may have had if you had been armed with your years of experience back then.

- The second exercise is a meditation that is frequently used in family systems therapy. In this meditation, as you sit quietly in a place where you will not be disturbed, imagine yourself as a child in the disturbing situation; also imagine that you are your adult self visiting your child self. Ask the younger version of yourself what they need from you. Maybe what she needs is for you to sit with her and rub her back. Or perhaps he needs you to show him how your life has changed. This process can be transformative and healing. We all have parts of ourselves that need healing, and this is a way to speak directly to those parts.

Examining Negative Thoughts

In step 2, we introduced you to cognitive distortions, or dysfunctional thoughts. Don't let the terminology confuse you—a negative thought is a negative thought is a negative thought. It's important to understand that some thoughts contain several distortions, making them even less reality-based. You may notice that during a depressive episode, your negative core beliefs about yourself come closer to the surface and trigger lots of negative thinking. As you know, the first step in learning how to manage negative thinking is to identify the negative thoughts themselves. As you learned in step 2, there are many types of cognitive distortions. Let's review them once more:

- Filtering
- Black-and-white thinking/ all-or-nothing thinking
- Overgeneralization
- Jumping to conclusions
- Catastrophizing
- Personalization
- Control fallacies

- Fallacy of fairness
- Blaming
- Shoulds
- Emotional reasoning
- Fallacy of change
- Labeling
- Always being right

If you need a refresher on the descriptions of these common types of negative thinking, flip back to pages 20 to 22. Once you know what something is, you can deal with it. When you recognize a thought being distorted, you are in a better position to reframe it. Negative thoughts or thought patterns have the potential to feel overwhelming, but they don't have to feel that way if you know how to identify them and know what to do when they arise. Let's take a look at some examples of negative thoughts and the cognitive distortions they are associated with. Then, on the following pages, we'll explore how to reframe them in a positive light.

"I'M SUCH A LOSER."

You had a job interview, but you didn't get the job. When you find out they hired someone else, your first thought is that you are a loser.

This negative thought primarily falls under the cognitive distortion of labeling, but it can also be personalization. Calling yourself names is not going to help you to move forward; rather, it will inevitably result in you feeling bad about yourself.

"THOSE PEOPLE ARE WHISPERING NEGATIVE THINGS ABOUT ME."

You're at the bank, and you see a group of people standing not too far away. They are whispering to one another, and one seems to glance in your direction. Your first thought is that they are saying something about you and you feel self-conscious and uncomfortable.

This negative thought primarily falls under the cognitive distortion of personalization, but it can also be jumping to conclusions. You assume these people are talking about you without any evidence.

"I'M A FAILURE AS A PARENT."

You had planned to take your kids to the park this Sunday afternoon, but you realize that there are things you must take care of around the house to prepare for the workweek ahead. You feel bad about it, and when your kids complain, your first thought is that you are failing as a parent.

This negative thought primarily falls under the cognitive distortion of emotional reasoning, but it can also be all-or-nothing thinking. Because you feel bad and guilty, you believe that this feeling *proves* that you did something wrong (and are therefore a failure).

"I SHOULD CALL MY SISTER."

You've been meaning to return your sister's call from earlier today, but you've been preoccupied with a big work project and even had to work through lunch. You look over at the phone and a feeling of guilt settles in your stomach; you think to yourself that you should call her back. You can't drop what you're doing, though, and you feel bad.

This negative thought falls under the cognitive distortion of shoulds. When you think to yourself that you *should* do something, it's because you feel that what you are doing instead is somehow wrong. This makes you feel unnecessarily guilty.

"I'M NEVER GOING TO BE ABLE TO DO THIS."

This morning, you set out to run five miles. However, after running four miles, you decide to turn around and go home; you're one mile short of your goal. On the way back, you think, "I'm never going to be able to run the whole five miles."

This negative thought falls under the cognitive distortion of black-and-white thinking or fortune-telling. Because you didn't make the five-mile goal you set for yourself this morning, you believe that you won't *ever* make it to five miles.

Reframing Negative Thoughts

Let's focus on reframing the thoughts in the previous section in a positive light. When reframing your thoughts, it's important to remember that you are *not* your thoughts; this is a crucial distinction to make when confronting them. It's also important that you make realistic statements when reframing your thoughts. You should not exaggerate or make anything up or even make things more positive than they really are. Just stick to the facts!

- "I'm such a loser."
  Reframe: "Another candidate was a better fit for that job than I was. I'll keep looking and going on interviews until I find the right fit for me."

- "Those people are whispering negative things about me."
  Reframe: "Those people are whispering to keep their conversation private. I have no idea what they are saying, and it's really not my business."

- "I'm a failure as a parent."
  Reframe: "I feel bad about canceling our trip to the park, but that doesn't make me a bad parent. In fact, I do a lot of great things with and for my kids."

- "I should call my sister."
  Reframe: "I'll make a note to return my sister's call as soon as I hand in this project."

- "I'm never going to be able to do this."
  Reframe: "I wasn't up to running five miles today. I ran four and that's more than I could run a year ago. I'll keep working toward my five-mile goal."

We hope you can see from these examples that negative thoughts can be managed by simply reframing them. You have more power than you think you do in taking control over your depression and improving your mood. A negative thought may seem louder and stronger than your ability to reframe it, but this just isn't true; your voice is impactful. You're gradually learning how to use your voice to talk back to those undermining thoughts. When your mind tells you that you're a failure, stand up to it.

"Stop it, and give yourself a chance."

—Dr. Aaron T. Beck

Identifying Your Negative Thoughts

With her own negative thinking patterns, Sarah has noticed that there are repeat offenders. Sometimes they just fade into the background when life gets busy, and she needs to remind herself what they are from time to time. She's found it helpful to write them down.

As you begin to really listen to your negative thoughts, have you noticed some repeat offenders that are common to you? What are your top five?

1. _____

2. _____

3. _____

4. _____

5. _____

Next, notice when you become triggered during negative thought patterns. Identify which cognitive distortion is associated with each of your five thoughts. Jot that down, too. As you engage in this exercise and others like it, you are gaining greater and greater awareness. Keep it up!

Other Constructive Ways to Cope with Negative Thinking

Your mind is powerful—it can convince you to hold false beliefs about yourself. You may feel frustrated, as if there's no way out. While your mind *is* a powerful tool, you can learn to work with it rather than letting it control you. As you proceed through this workbook, you are learning that negative thoughts can be reframed or transformed into positive ones. Aren't you glad to know you're not stuck with a negative mind-set?

Using the tools in this chapter, you can observe a negative thought, acknowledge it, identify it for what it is, reframe it, and then create a positive mind-set. You are doing the work here, and you're going to see firsthand that you have the power to change this myopic pattern of negative thinking. Following are some more helpful suggestions for dealing with your negative thoughts and reclaiming your power.

QUESTION THE VALIDITY OF NEGATIVE THOUGHTS

Negative thoughts are bound to come into your mind. What you do with them is up to you. Take a moment and assess whether these thoughts have any truth to them. What would you say if a good friend told you that she felt this way about herself? Sometimes it's easier to help other people before being kind to yourself. After you imagine what you'd say to a close friend, use that viewpoint on yourself. You're probably being unnecessarily hard on yourself because negative thoughts have a way of pushing us to act that way toward ourselves; it's often called a "double-standard" technique. You can fight back with logic as opposed to emotional reasoning. That's why we question the validity of these thoughts. For example, is there any evidence to support the idea that you are truly a bad person? If this was a court of law and you were an attorney, how would you cross-examine the thought?

TREAT YOUR NEGATIVE THOUGHTS
LIKE A MISBEHAVING CHILD

Dr. Adrian Wells discusses how to deal with negative thoughts by using the "recalcitrant child" metaphor in his book *Metacognitive Therapy for Anxiety and Depression*. Imagine that a child is misbehaving in a store. In order to discourage the child's poor behavior, the best course of action is to keep an eye on the child but ignore the behavior itself. Your negative thoughts are similar to the badly behaved child. You know that they're there, but you don't need to engage with them. Be mindfully aware of the thoughts while staying detached.

BE KIND TO YOURSELF

You've already got these pervasive negative thoughts, which lead to bad feelings. What makes those feelings worse is when you judge yourself for feeling the way that you feel. Your feelings are real, and you have a right to feel them. Sarah has often wondered what it would be like if she didn't deal with depression. She has thought about other people around her who appear to be "happy." Her mom has a mantra that helps her cope with these thoughts: "Compare and despair." This concept is tied to the cognitive distortion of jumping to conclusions. You aren't a mind reader; you can't know what other people are thinking or feeling. If you try to guess, you'll find yourself making assumptions that may or may not be true. The only way to know what someone is thinking is to ask.

Making judgments about yourself and making comparisons with others will lead to further feelings of shame and disappointment. Try to let go of what thinking these thoughts "means." They don't mean anything in the objective sense. They are just thoughts that are irritating and taking up space in your mind. The way you feel is the way you are feeling right now. It's not forever, even though you might think it will be that way. You'll get through this no matter what, but you can reduce your suffering if you can accept these thoughts and release judgment on them. Observe the thought with a nonjudgmental stance, and then either practice letting go of it or reframing it the best that you can without judgment—whichever works best for you.

PRACTICE GRATITUDE

When Sarah was feeling down, her mom used to encourage her to make a list of 10 things that she was grateful for. It helped her to see that there were good things in her life that she was forgetting while in the throes of depression; there *were* things in her life that contributed to her happiness. She learned that recognizing what she has rather than what she doesn't helps lift her feelings of sadness. You'll see that this can be true for you, too. We'll talk more about gratitude in step 10, but for now, in the space that follows, list 10 things you are grateful for:

1. ~~Friends~~ ~~cool + warm place living retired benefits~~
2. ~~_____~~
3. _____
4. _____
5. _____
6. _____
7. _____
8. _____
9. _____
10. _____

REMEMBER YOUR STRENGTHS

Too often we focus on our flaws rather than acknowledge our strengths. While it's helpful to see where you can improve, you also need to focus on what you're good at. Seeing the positive within yourself helps you combat your negative thinking. You do have value, and acknowledging what you're skilled at will help you understand that. Here's your chance to give yourself a shout-out. Reflect on what you're proud of about yourself. What are you good at? We realize that for people dealing with depression, this can be challenging due to their automatic thoughts. Try your best to find some things that you are proud of, no matter how big or small. In the space that follows, list your top 10 positive qualities:

1. _____

2. _____

3. _____

4. _____

5. _____

6. _____

7. _____

8. _____

9. _____

10. _____

SPEAK TO A MENTAL HEALTH PROFESSIONAL

If you feel that your negative thinking is too difficult to cope with on your own, consider seeing a psychologist or other mental health professional with expertise in CBT and/or treatment of depression. Along with the strategies in this workbook, they can provide you with tools, support, and guidance. Speaking with a qualified professional can be an important step in your healing journey.

Applying ACT to Cope with Negative Thinking

Fighting your negative thoughts can feel exhausting. Reframe this idea of being in battle with your thoughts in a positive way. Cognitive defusion (deliteralization) is a strategy to help you view your thoughts for what they are as opposed to what they appear to be. When you use defusion, you are paying close attention to your thoughts and how they influence your actions. Here are three ACT-based strategies to defuse negative thinking:

1. **REWORD THE THOUGHT SO IT DOESN'T HAVE TO DO WITH YOU PERSONALLY, BUT WITH THE ACTION.** For example, you might think, "I'm going to look stupid at this party." Change the thought to, "I'm having the thought that I'll look stupid at this party." This distances you from the thought and focuses on the thought as external to yourself.

2. **FIND THE HUMOR IN A NEGATIVE THOUGHT BY SINGING IT TO THE TUNE OF A SILLY SONG.** Let's say you're thinking, "I am a failure." Sing the thought aloud to the tune of "My Darling Clementine." Hearing the thought sung out loud will lessen the harsh impact it has on you.

3. **RECOGNIZE THAT SOME THOUGHTS REAPPEAR AS ONGOING CHARACTERS IN YOUR "BRAIN STORY."** Observe the thought entering your mind and acknowledge that it's making another appearance. It's like that annoying neighbor who has a tendency to show up unannounced—and uninvited. You remember him, of course; it's no surprise that he's here. Politely escort him out of the house. And do the same for your repetitive thoughts.

Truths to Remember about Negative Thinking

Negative thinking can become a way of life; it's a mentality that develops over time. The pattern can be broken, but it will take time. Our brains are malleable, so with some hard work, you can have a less pessimistic view of yourself, the world, and your future and, as a result, modify your feelings and actions. That's your ultimate goal, and you're working diligently to get there. As you make an effort to reframe your thoughts, you're bound to hit mental roadblocks. That's okay. Just keep going and focus on your goal: To learn to cope with negative thinking over time.

Negative thoughts have a way of taking up residence in your brain, but they didn't sign a lease, and so do not have the right to dwell there. Remember these truths:

- Overcoming negative thinking takes time.

- Negative thoughts can feel overpowering.

- It can feel uncomfortable to examine thoughts that are connected to your sense of self.

- Don't force yourself to think positively. Instead, think realistically.

- Do what comes naturally when addressing thoughts (e.g., mindfully accepting versus reframing).

- Negative core beliefs often develop early and are stubborn.

- Changing behavior is just as important as changing the thought itself. In fact, often by changing behavior, you can change your thoughts! So take the thought and use it as an opportunity to modify the way you act toward yourself and others.

Review

In this chapter, you became even more familiar with the nature of negative thoughts. Knowing how to match your negative thoughts to cognitive distortions goes a long way in helping you recognize them for what they are: untruths and misperceptions. We also touched on the concept of negative core beliefs as the basis for our negative thoughts. That's okay if you didn't identify any, because you don't necessarily need to know the exact cause of your negative thoughts to be able to use your newly developing skills to tame them. The next step is going to take you even deeper, as we'll be discussing specific ways to directly target negative thinking. In the meantime, think about what this chapter has illuminated for you, and write about it here:

Change neg thoughts to positive

Homework

For the next few days, carry a pencil and a pad with you that you can access at any time. (You can also use a notes app on your smartphone.) Throughout the day, write down any negative thoughts that come to you. Notice any repeat offenders and mark an asterisk next to them. Then return to this workbook. Write down all of those thoughts here:

_____

_____

_____

_____

_____

_____

_____

_____

_____

_____

_____

_____

Once you've written down the thoughts, you can practice reframing them. You can also try the other suggestions, too, like singing them to the tune of a silly song.

Remember those repeat offenders you marked with an asterisk? Those are the thoughts you are going to focus on more deeply as we move on to the strategies that challenge negative thinking in step 6.

Break Negative Thought Patterns

You've made amazing progress. As you've moved through this workbook step-by-step, you've been gathering clues and gaining skills that are part of the detailed plan to curb your negative thinking, which we'll cover in this chapter.

> *"Worry and obsession get worse when you try to control your thoughts."*
>
> —Dr. Judith Beck

A basic ingredient in step 6 is this: Do not try to *stop* your negative thoughts (see the sidebar on page 77). This may sound counterintuitive, because you want to be able to change your thoughts. But the way to change negative thinking is to acknowledge the thoughts and work with them rather than fight them. You've heard the expression, "If you can't beat 'em, join 'em." That's a great way to think about how to deal with your negative thought patterns. You'll be able to successfully change your thoughts if you recognize them and reframe them the way you've been practicing, and then move on. Let's get to work on this step now.

A Close Look at Creating Thought Records

In step 3, we introduced you to thought records and showed you how to visualize your negative thought processes. You learned that when you see your distorted thinking, you're better able to confront and deal with it. Now let's go over the specific steps involved in creating a thought record so that you can become adept at this process.

The following five steps lead you on a fascinating journey from acknowledging the negative thought to changing it to something positive. If you'd like to give this a try right now, you can respond to these questions on the thought-record worksheet on page 85. Or you can just read through them and fill out your thought record later.

1. **The situation and the emotion.** Describe in detail where you were, what happened, and how you felt.

2. **Negative thought.** What was the first thought that entered your mind? Try not to think too hard about this—just write what popped into your head so you can put a spotlight on your automatic thought. As an aside: What are the benefits of changing negative thinking? Some answers might be: "I'll feel better about myself," "My relationships will improve," "I'll be able to let go of things instead of obsessing about them," "My quality of life will be better," or "I'll feel happy more often." Also consider the following:

- Which cognitive distortions are you using in your automatic thought? (See pages 20 to 22 for a refresher.) These happen when your brain is on autopilot. They aren't part of you, and you don't need to feel guilty for having them.

- If you can, trace the automatic thought back to the first time you had it. As discussed in step 5, these thoughts tend to relate to a negative core belief that developed during childhood. Once you find the origin of the thought, question if this thought has helped you or hurt you from the past up until now. How has the thought served you? Is there any benefit to having it? What are the costs if you continue to think that way?

3. **Evidence that does and does not support that thought.** Reality-test your automatic thought. Put that thought on trial. What evidence do you have to support this thought? If you were speaking with a friend having the same thought, what would you say to them? Also, what evidence do you have the supports an entirely different way of thinking? What's in it for you if you do?

4. **Alternative thoughts.** You've got a hold on your negative thought now. It's time to confront it and mold it into something more realistic—in other words, reframe it. Think of the thought as a giant piece of clay. Your thought, just like clay, is malleable. You can change the way you view this situation. How can you think about this incident differently so that it doesn't contain any cognitive distortions and passes the reality test? Are you still wrapped up in thinking negatively? Do your best, and your thinking will change in time. Remember, this is a process. You may have been thinking negatively for the majority of your life, so this is a pattern that will take some time to break. You can do this!

5. **Emotion.** Check in with yourself. What are you feeling now? Chances are after having put your thoughts out in the light throughout this process, you feel some relief, and that's great!

A REALISTIC-THINKING PLAN

Create a mantra or short saying that reminds you to think in a more realistic way. This mantra will serve to remind you that you *can* change the way you think. Here are some examples of possible mantras: *I am not my thoughts, I've got this, I deserve to be well, I am helping myself right now, I believe in myself,* and *I will be kind to myself.* You can create your own positive affirmation and let it guide you into a healthier everyday mind-set. Write your own mantra here:

Inevitably, though, there will be times in your life where you'll backslide into negative thinking. It's not your fault. We all have automatic thoughts that get the best of us. The important thing is to have a plan so that you'll know what to do. Let's say "I'm a loser" pops into your head. Remember that you have a tendency to label yourself with unkind names and "defuse" from the thought by saying, "I'm having a thought that I'm a loser." Then say your mantra. Go through the process of creating a thought record if your mantra isn't enough to guide you back toward a positive thought process. Remember, this is your plan and you are in the driver's seat, so do whatever works for you.

A study conducted by Stanford University showed that people who spent 90 minutes a day in nature had a significantly decreased incidence of depression. It may be difficult to get yourself out of the house some days, but with nature waiting right outside your door to nurture you, give yourself a little push, put on your shoes, open the door, and step outside. We bet you'll be glad you did.

Thought Record Worksheet

SITUATION:
EMOTION:

NEGATIVE AUTOMATIC THOUGHT:	EVIDENCE THAT SUPPORTS THE THOUGHT:	EVIDENCE THAT DOES NOT SUPPORT THE THOUGHT:

ALTERNATIVE THOUGHTS:
EMOTION:

SITUATION:
EMOTION:

NEGATIVE AUTOMATIC THOUGHT:	EVIDENCE THAT SUPPORTS THE THOUGHT:	EVIDENCE THAT DOES NOT SUPPORT THE THOUGHT:

ALTERNATIVE THOUGHTS:
EMOTION:

Helpful Ways to Enhance Objective Thinking in the Moment

When you're stuck in a negative thought cycle, it can be hard to find an immediate way out of it. Here are some helpful tips to help you take control and think more rationally on the spot:

BRAINSTORM THROUGH WRITING. If you just can't get past a negative thought, write about it in a journal using a free-association technique—that is, write whatever comes to mind without editing or critiquing. You may be surprised by the insight you gain.

BE IN THE MOMENT AND BREATHE. Practicing mindfulness (being in the moment) is an important skill to have in general, so we'll discuss it in-depth when we get to step 10. For now, bring your attention to the present moment and try to observe whatever you're experiencing without judging it. Try this exercise: Breathe in on the count of five, feeling your diaphragm expand. Hold on to the breath for a moment, and then breathe out. Continue this process for a while. Breathing like this grounds you and helps you stay in the moment.

FOCUS ON THE PEOPLE YOU LOVE. There are people in your life who care about you. When Sarah brings to mind the people she loves and who love her, her mood improves. Instead of focusing on whatever negative thought is hassling you, think about the people you care about and the qualities you love about them. Your mind may attempt to convince you that no one cares about you. Prove it wrong by reaching out to those who do love you, so that you can reaffirm that they are out there and they care.

ACCEPT THAT YOU ARE FALLIBLE. Acknowledging your humanity and the fact that you make mistakes is a simple yet profound realization. When we imagine ourselves as perfect beings, we will be disappointed when we do something that we feel is less than perfect. Remind yourself that you will make many mistakes throughout your life. This is okay because it is part of life. No one is perfect.

CELEBRATE. If something good happened during the day, acknowledge it and celebrate it. There are so many wonderful moments in our lives, and if we don't acknowledge them, we will stop recognizing them. For example, did someone compliment you on your outfit? Give yourself a little cheer! Something that may seem small, like a compliment or even a bright smile from a passerby, is meaningful and worthy of celebration.

MINDFULLY DETACH FROM YOUR THOUGHTS. Instead of wrestling with the negative thought and trying to ignore it in hopes that it will go away, observe it as if it is a scrolling marquee sign where the words change frequently. Your thoughts are not stationary; they come and they go. See them as external from you, rather than as part of you.

REMIND YOURSELF THAT EVERYTHING PASSES. As a teen, Sarah didn't know what her mom meant when she said, "Everything passes." Now that Sarah is older, she understands that while certain aspects of life might seem overwhelming or depressing right now, they will change. Nothing stays the same, and thank goodness it doesn't! Depression doesn't last forever and it's important to remind yourself of that when you're feeling down. This feeling is temporary. And if you continue to do the work in this book, you can expedite the process of feeling better.

KNOW THAT THERE IS A SOLUTION. You may not be able to see it right now, but there is a solution to whatever problem you're worrying about. Those negative thoughts are telling you that everything is hopeless and you should just give up; you're not going to find a way out of this situation. Those thoughts are wrong. You *will* find the answer; it just might take some time. Worrying about the problem won't get you any closer to finding that answer. What will help you find a solution? Focus on the facts, reframe your negative thoughts, take productive action, and keep going by whatever means necessary.

Ongoing Exercises for Mood Enhancement

You can support the CBT work you've been doing, such as creating thought records and examining cognitive distortions, with a few tangible activities you can do on a regular basis that enhance positive thinking. From exercising and doing an art project to meditating and listening to music, you have many additional options for enhancing your mood. Place a check mark alongside the entries in the following sections to indicate which of these you would like to incorporate into your life on a regular basis.

☐ WORK OUT

According to the Mayo Clinic, exercising for 30 minutes a day three to five days a week may significantly improve the symptoms of depression. When you exercise, your brain releases "happy chemicals" called endorphins, which may ease depression. After checking with your doctor, start with 20 minutes of cardio a couple of times a week to get those feel-good brain chemicals flowing. Brisk walking is a great place to start. When you exercise regularly, you'll notice that you are starting to feel good physically, which helps you feel better mentally and emotionally.

☐ MEDITATE

According to a study by Barbara Fredrickson, a professor of psychology at the University of North Carolina at Chapel Hill, people who practiced meditation on a daily basis experienced more positive thinking than people who didn't have this practice. Additionally, the same people who meditated saw positive long-term effects in their lives, such as better overall mood and focus. If you don't know how to meditate, there are many resources online, in bookstores, and maybe even in your community. Go explore and consider starting a practice.

Drawing Your Negative Thoughts

Along the lines of using creativity to improve your mood, here's an exercise you can try to help transform a negative thought into a less troubling one. In the space below, write down the negative thought. Next to that, draw a picture of what that thought might look like if it were an animal, a person, or an object. Maybe it's a monster with five heads. Whatever you imagine it to look like is perfectly valid.

Below your depiction of the negative thought, write another thought that changes your negative thought in any way you want. Next to the reframed thought, draw a picture of what *that* thought might look like as an animal, a person, or an object.

When you've completed the drawings, compare them to each other. What's different? Which do you like better? This is a fun visual representation of what it's like to creatively reframe your thinking.

☐ LISTEN TO MUSIC

Music soothes the body and soul and has been used therapeutically for millennia. When Sarah is feeling depressed, she listens to music she finds uplifting and starts to feel better. Choose songs or musical pieces that you know elevate your mood and listen often.

☐ DO SOMETHING CREATIVE

Being creative can be therapeutic. Whether that means drawing, acting, writing, or making pottery, you're free to express yourself in any way you choose. You don't have to be an artist to have fun creating something. The process itself is enjoyable, but when you've created something, you'll also be able to see and feel the effects of that creative process, either through basking in a sense of accomplishment or admiring your handiwork. Check out the drawing exercise on page 89.

☐ "ACT AS IF"

"Act as if" is a commonly used strategy within CBT. It's along the same lines as "Fake it till you make it." What these sayings mean is that even if you don't feel a certain way, act as though you do. For example, are you afraid to walk into an unfamiliar setting? No one needs to know that you're nervous. Hold your head high and stroll into the new situation as if you have all the confidence you need.

When you keep "acting as if," eventually you won't be acting anymore. And the same goes for thinking positively. You might have to work very hard at it right now because you're working diligently to break your negative-thinking habit, but the more you go through the motions of using your CBT skills, the more familiar you'll become with this new way of thinking. And before you know it, curbing your negative thoughts will feel like a part of your routine.

How Do You Stay Positive?

We've covered several ideas and exercises for maintaining a more objective outlook in this chapter. Have you tried some of them? Are you planning to? Maybe you have some ideas of your own that we didn't cover here. There's a lot to work with in this chapter, so reflect on the things that help *you* get or stay positive—or at least those things you think might help. List them in the following space. Remember, this list is unique and personal to you. No two lists are going to be the same because no two human beings are the same. So, what helps you stay upbeat? What are some of the ideas you plan to try out?

_____

_____

_____

_____

_____

_____

_____

_____

According to the Mayo Clinic, positive thinking can help reduce stress and improve the ability to cope with life's obstacles. It may also have several other health benefits, including a longer life, less incidence of depression, greater immunity, and less heart disease.

Review

Breaking negative thought patterns is what step 6 is all about, so in this chapter, you've been armed with a number of exercises to help you break the pattern of negative thinking, both in the long term and in the moment. We often don't realize how distorted and negative our thoughts are until we begin to pay attention and record them on a thought record worksheet. This allows you to transform them into healthier and more rational thoughts, shifting our perspective from negativity to objectivity. This is what makes the CBT approach to dealing with depression so great at transforming people's lives for the better. What has this chapter illuminated for you? Write about it here:

When you have these negative thoughts Go to your
Mantra 1st, then evaluate the thought by acting it
Do some deep breathing to re establish yourself
May draw a picture of that thought
#1 Be mindful Think of £1 love + how they treat you
Breathe accept you are not perfect
Remind self "This too shall pass" Know I is a way
to work it out   Meditate + work out both
to priorities

Homework

For the next week, fill out a thought record if your mind goes down a negative path. Try to do this several times a day to really bring your negative thoughts into the light. Also use your personal mantra often to keep yourself thinking objectively. Then, at the end of the week, write about your experience. Did you notice a shift in your mood? Even a subtle one? Did you gravitate toward one particular cognitive distortion? Reflect here:

_____

_____

_____

_____

_____

_____

Did you find that you tend to catastrophize a lot? Maybe one of the other cognitive distortions is more your habit (or maybe you struggle with multiple distortions). Start thinking about where this type of distorted thinking comes from. If you are prone to catastrophizing, take a moment to remember a time in your early life when you thought something terrible was going to happen. Did it happen? Now write about what it is that you're worried will happen. Compare the two scenarios. What do these two situations have in common?

_____

_____

_____

_____

_____

_____

Look at the list of things on pages 86 to 87 to help you stay objective. Incorporate one of those techniques this week to see if it brightens your outlook. What effect did it have?

7/8/23 Exercise helps

Don't Procrastinate

For someone with depression, a small task can be perceived as incredibly difficult to accomplish. For this reason, among others, procrastination can be a real issue when you are depressed. Some people mistake a lack of motivation for laziness, but generally when people procrastinate, it isn't because they are lazy; it's because they feel stuck. It may be hard to begin a task when you feel down and are being plagued by thoughts like "What's the point?" We promise you that there is a point. In this chapter, we'll help you look past the negative thought patterns that are telling you to put things off, do them tomorrow, or not do them at all. Step 7 is all about how to manage your tasks to get things done. Are you ready? Let's go!

Common Causes of Procrastination, Plus Remedies

Procrastination isn't only a problem for people with depression. Virtually everyone procrastinates from time to time. Maybe we put something off because we are afraid we won't be able to conquer it. Maybe we're thinking we need to do it "perfectly." Or perhaps we think the task will take "forever." These are some of the common reasons why we procrastinate. But let's focus on some potential reasons why you personally might be procrastinating. It's not that you don't *want* to get it done; it just might feel like you *can't* for a variety of reasons. Let's see how you can push back against the common causes of procrastination and get the task done while dealing with your depression.

ABSENCE OF ROUTINE

Some of us have trouble creating a routine, whereas others have an inherent sense of organization. Don't punish yourself if routine and structure don't come naturally to you. We all have strengths and challenges. If you struggle to stay on task or create a routine, ask a friend who is more organized to help. There are also many resources online that help with task management.

Because Sarah had trouble staying on track, she searched for a technique to keep her focused. She created the Get It Done routine we are sharing here. It's based on a time-management method called the Pomodoro Technique. You can use Sarah's Get It Done routine whether you are in an office or working from home by following these three steps:

1. Set your timer for 20 minutes and work on your task until the timer goes off.

2. Set your timer for 5 minutes and take a 5-minute break. Look over what you've done or get up, take a walk, meditate—anything that calms you.

3. Repeat steps 1 and 2 three more times, so that you've had four 20-minute sessions of work and four 5-minute breaks.

This routine is under two hours, which isn't a lot of time, but we guarantee you will have made noticeable progress on your task. Now, choose something that you've been procrastinating doing, and use the next two hours to make some headway. After those two hours, come back here. What were some of the positive effects of using the Get It Done routine? What were some of the challenges? What did you do during your breaks? How did this method help you stop procrastinating?

_____

_____

_____

_____

_____

_____

_____

When we are working on a computer, it can be tempting to deviate from what we are doing to check social media. Sarah knows that she sometimes struggles with the impulse to check her newsfeed. To stay focused and on task, we recommend not having social media tabs open. Better yet, use some free time management software (e.g., freedom.to) to temporarily block access to those sites. Set aside a specific time to catch up on social media.

A TASK YOU DON'T WANT TO DO

There may be some items on your to-do list that you honestly just aren't motivated to do. In that category may be things like compiling your paperwork for your taxes, cleaning the house, doing yard work, and so on. One of the reasons these tasks seem unpleasant is that they feel overwhelming. In this case, try breaking down a task that you don't want to do into smaller parts.

You don't have to do it all at once. Think about it: If you have a plate of food in front of you, do you shove all the food in your mouth at once? That would be really unpleasant and result in you feeling physically ill. You eat one bite of food at a time—first a bite of the salmon, then a bite of the broccoli, and then a bite of the rice. (Yeah, we tend to eat pretty healthy.) So, let's practice.

Pick a task that overwhelms you and break it down into about 10 steps. For example, let's say cleaning the house is on your to-do list, but you've been procrastinating. You can break a task like this down into smaller steps, such as "vacuum/sweep all the rooms," then "dust all the rooms" and so on. Or you could clean the house one room at a time—for example, "clean the living room," then "clean the kitchen." You can break these tasks down even further. For instance, in the living room, one step could be "clear off the coffee table." In the kitchen, a step might be "clean the stove top." When you've listed the steps of your chosen task here, try doing at least the first two on the list. You may then find that you're on a roll.

_____

_____

_____

_____

_____

_____

_____

THINKING IT WILL TAKE TOO LONG

One reason we avoid doing a task is because we think it is going to "take forever." It may be difficult to see the light at the end of the task tunnel. If you've been practicing Sarah's Get It Done routine and breaking down your unwanted task into smaller steps, you'll start to believe that things can get done in a reasonable amount of time. However, the distorted thought that something will "take forever" is still likely to come up. In reality, nothing takes your entire life to complete except your life itself.

Using the list you created in the previous section, estimate how long each step would take you to complete or create a new breakdown for a different task.

Realistically estimating how long something will take assures you that it won't really take "forever." With any long-term goal, you'll get there in time if you approach it in a series of tangible steps. Estimate the time needed for your task here:

_____

_____

_____

_____

_____

_____

_____

_____

FEELING ANXIOUS

When we feel anxious about doing a good job on the task ahead of us, we tend to avoid doing it. Of course, you can now turn to your CBT skills in order to help get your tasks done, but it's important to note that this tendency to avoid anxiety-provoking tasks is true for a lot of people. Here's an example that might resonate: You avoid getting out of bed when your alarm goes off because you feel anxious about everything you have to get done that day; you fear you won't do it perfectly or correctly, or even worse, you'll fail completely.

When the idea of not performing perfectly or messing something up causes you anxiety and leads to procrastination, just tell yourself that you'll do the best you can do. Often when you take the first step, anxiety starts to decrease. If you can push yourself to take an action, you'll see what happens to your anxiety. Once you get going, your anxiety will usually lessen. Another tool you can use is to find a mantra that reminds you that you are doing the best you can in this moment. Maybe it's as simple as, "I'm doing the best that I can in this moment." Sarah's friend Maggie May Ethridge gave her a great mantra: "I'm focusing on what I'm doing, not on how I am feeling." So take a lesson from Maggie May and focus on what you are doing this very moment. All you need to do is what you are doing—even if that's as simple as swinging your legs over the bed and standing up to face the day.

What sort of tasks tend to cause you anxiety? What is a mantra you can use to help you focus on the present and not on the outcome so that you can keep going and accomplish your task?

_____

_____

_____

_____

_____

_____

_____

NOT BELIEVING IN YOURSELF

When you are feeling depressed, it's easy to fall into the habit of self-doubt. When you feel unsure about your ability to do something or you believe that you can't do it, procrastination is much more likely to surface. It's okay to feel doubtful about your abilities. It's what you do with that feeling that matters, though.

Here's a great way to cope with those "I can't do this" thoughts. Remember a time when you were afraid you couldn't do something, but you did it anyway. Here's an example from Sarah's life: When it was time for Sarah to go to college, she didn't believe she could cope with her chronic anxiety on her own at school; she was terrified to leave her parents. Her first thought was to procrastinate. A year off between high school and college sounded like a good plan. However, she knew that putting it off wouldn't get her closer to her goal of an undergraduate degree, and she pushed herself to attend college. Now, when Sarah feels like she can't do something, she reminds herself of that monumental choice she made in which she triumphed over her own self-doubt. She believed in herself, and you can, too.

Take a moment to recall a time when you didn't think you could accomplish something, but you did despite your self-doubt. We've all had those moments, and whether they are big or small, they matter. If you're depressed and coping with cognitive distortions that affect your ability to see your accomplishments clearly, ask for an outside perspective on your achievements. It's okay to ask for help if you're having difficulty pinpointing your accomplishments. In the space that follows, write about a time in your life when you were able to work through a feeling of insecurity and get your task done:

_____

_____

_____

_____

_____

_____

Rewards for Accomplishing a Task

Ice cream is one of Sarah's favorite desserts. Her kids love it, too, and even though they'd gladly eat it for breakfast, she reminds them that it's an end-of-day treat. In her home, ice cream is a reward for having eaten a healthy dinner.

The concept of rewards can also be applied to task management. When you go through the steps you've set for yourself and then ultimately complete the task, find a way to reward yourself—as we know from behaviorism (remember Pavlov and his salivating dogs?), tasks followed by a favorable outcome tend to be strengthened. Here are a few ideas:

- Go out with a friend
- Drink a milkshake
- Play a video game
- Listen to a podcast
- Watch a TV show
- Order dinner instead of cooking

- Dance like no one's watching
- Catch up on social media
- Work on a hobby
- Read a book or magazine
- Take a bubble bath

The list of rewards is virtually endless. What gives you joy? Reward yourself with that when you've accomplished your task—you deserve it! In the following space, make a list of some rewards you can give yourself when you achieve your goal:

_____

_____

_____

_____

_____

_____

Questioning Perfectionism

As we've mentioned, a common reason for procrastinating is that you're concerned about not doing whatever you're facing "perfectly." The reality is that perfectionism will prevent you from starting the task. You'll likely agonize over the task. Perfec-

"Have no fear of perfection—you'll never reach it."

—Salvador Dalí

tionism is a symptom of the cognitive distortion black-and-white thinking (if you need a reminder, see page 20). With this negative thought, either you will do it perfectly or you will be a complete failure. The fear of failure is a major obstacle; therefore, you'll need to work on reframing the idea of doing

something "perfectly" or "correctly." To reframe this idea, ask yourself if you will do the best you can. If the answer is yes, which we're sure it will be, then you can feel confident enough to get started.

Let's say you feel overwhelmed because you want to clean your garage. Old boxes are stacked everywhere, the shelves are jam-packed, the floor is filthy, and so on. In other words, it's a garage. But you have a vision of a spotless, organized garage. You don't want to clean the garage because if it isn't perfect when you're done, you know you'll feel defeated. What if you made a goal to go through the stacks of boxes instead? This weekend, you'll tackle the boxes, next weekend the shelves, and so on until your garage is as clean as a garage can be. Acknowledge that it will never be spotless. No one is watching over you or taking notes about how clean your garage is.

Do you have an unrealistic idea of how something should be? Do you avoid doing the laundry because there's always going to be more laundry and you'll never have a perfectly empty laundry room or hamper? That's just a simple example, of course, but try to apply this line of reasoning to why you may be procrastinating. In the space that follows, jot down some tasks that daunt you because you want to do them perfectly. Once you've done that, record how you might change the way you think about those things and encourage yourself to let go of the idea of perfection:

_____

_____

_____

_____

_____

_____

_____

_____

MISTAKES ARE OPPORTUNITIES TO GROW

You *can* stop procrastinating when you acknowledge that you are fallible and therefore will make mistakes in life. Maybe you're writing a report for work, but you forget to save the document and lose a paragraph you were proud of. It's not the end of the world. Here's an opportunity to get more creative and write something even better. We realize you might be tempted to yell at the computer or punch a pillow. That's okay. We all feel frustrated from time to time, so it's perfectly normal and acceptable if you need to step away to collect yourself. And if you have to punch the occasional pillow out of frustration, that's okay, too. You're not hurting anyone. The same goes for yelling at your computer, since it doesn't have feelings. (Or, at least not yet!) Just be sure to follow the golden rule of not doing harm—to yourself, to others, or to any property. Plus, odds are you will feel a sense of empowerment when you take a positive action to help yourself move forward. It might take a moment to get back on task, so give yourself permission to take that time to collect yourself.

Mistakes are lessons and opportunities to grow as a person. Perfectionism is often associated with being afraid of failing, but all you can do is what you're doing—keep working on your task and moving forward. The fear of failure does not have to paralyze you. Mistakes are simply a part of life, and it's how you respond to those mishaps that matters. You can feel bad about them and stop working on your task, or you can remind yourself that everyone makes mistakes and forgive yourself. You'll feel better if you choose option two.

Now it's your turn to reflect on a mistake that you've made. Think of a time when you made a mistake as well as how you overcame that blunder and kept going. Write about this moment to encourage yourself that you survived a mistake.

_____

_____

_____

_____

_____

_____

_____

_____

_____

_____

_____

Why Perfectionism Doesn't Work

Some people might think that it's perfectly fine to strive for perfection. But when perfection is in your sight and things don't go as planned, it can feel downright debilitating and exacerbate the symptoms of depression. If you need more convincing to let your idea of perfection go in order to accomplish a task that's been on your to-do list, here it is:

- **PERFECTIONISM TRICKS YOU INTO BELIEVING YOU AREN'T "GOOD ENOUGH."** This is an illusion. You don't have to report to anyone but yourself. Tell yourself that you are working as hard as you can when you start to think that things need to be perfect. Fight against this concept of "perfect" by reminding yourself that you're trying hard and that counts.

- **PERFECTIONISM MAKES PEOPLE FEEL STRESSED-OUT.** It can contribute to high levels of depression and anxiety and lead to avoidance. Remember that this workbook is here to remind you that you can get through depression. One of the ways to help you do that is to reject perfectionism as a way of avoiding doing what you have to do.

- **PERFECTIONISM CAN IMPACT THE QUALITY OF YOUR WORK.** You will procrastinate more because you don't want to do it "wrong." You may put more pressure on yourself by waiting until the last minute to do something because of this fear.

- **PERFECTIONISM MAY ENCOURAGE YOU TO FOCUS ON THE NEGATIVE RATHER THAN ON THE POSITIVE ASPECTS OF WHAT YOU'RE DOING.** In reality, you are doing productive tasks. Perfectionism will cause you to forget the good things you're doing for yourself. Remind yourself of the positive things you're doing when you start to go into a perfectionist mode of thinking.

- **PERFECTIONISM MIGHT RESULT IN YOU MISSING OUT ON SOME EXCITING OPPORTUNITIES.** When you're open to achieving a goal, you'll see more ways to make that happen. Let go of perfectionism and notice the creative solutions in front of you that you wouldn't have seen otherwise.

Review

This chapter put a spotlight on procrastination, illuminating its negative impact, and it familiarized you with some of its common causes, as well as how to challenge them and create solutions. We also discussed how to break down a big task into smaller steps so that it doesn't feel so overwhelming. You learned Sarah's Get It Done routine, which helps you accomplish a task in short increments, and hopefully you've already started putting it to good use. We also helped you identify some things you can reward yourself with when you complete your task. Since perfectionism plays such a big role in procrastination, we spent a good deal of time discussing why it doesn't have to stop you from doing what you need to do. Now you have the tools to combat procrastination, no matter the cause! What has this chapter illuminated for you? Write about it here:

_____

_____

_____

_____

_____

_____

_____

_____

_____

_____

_____

Homework

This week, pay attention to when you are tempted to procrastinate. When you start to put something off, record the task here and break down that task into a series of steps as you learned to do earlier in this chapter. Also estimate how long each step will take and write that next to each step.

_____

_____

_____

_____

_____

_____

_____

_____

_____

_____

_____

_____

_____

Do the first item on your list using the Get It Done routine. If you're starting to feel bogged down by the idea that what you're doing needs to be perfect, think about how you can view the task differently and then move forward. When you've taken all the steps, no matter how long it takes, reward yourself with a special treat.

Activate Your Behavior and Face Your Fears

In the previous chapter, we discussed ways to stop procrastinating. Now we're going to delve into methods that will help you change your behavioral patterns— the *B* in *CBT*. The most important message to take from this step is that your behavior has the power to impact your mood just as much as your thoughts do. Behavioral activation (BA), which capitalizes on this fact, involves first seeing this in action and then gradually increasing behaviors that you can predict will help improve your mood. In other words, in this aspect of CBT, you learn to change your behavior, which in turn helps lift your mood.

B is for *Behavior*

CBT theory states that all of our experiences can be framed within a triangle, featuring thoughts, feelings, and actions in the corners. Imagine the corners of this triangle are connected to one another with arrows that can point in either direction, symbolizing the fact that each corner is capable of influencing the other two. In other words, how we *think* influences how we *feel* and how we *act*; but how we *act* also influences how we *feel* and *think*; and finally, how we *feel* influences how we *think* and *act*. All three are equally important and all influence one another. In addition, because they are all connected, *if you change one, the other two will also change.* So if you don't like the way you feel, you have two good options: (1) change how you think or (2) change how you act. A lot

> *"The most difficult thing is the decision to act, the rest is merely tenacity. The fears are paper tigers. You can do anything you decide to do. You can act to change and control your life; and the procedure, the process is its own reward."*
>
> —Amelia Earhart

of research has been done on the behavioral (i.e., action) part of the triangle, with results that appear to be as good as the cognitive (i.e., thought) portion of the triangle. The main idea behind BA is that when people feel depressed, they decrease the activities they would normally participate in, and this limits their access to the things they normally do that serve as mood boosters. One of the key things that maintains depression is inertia. Behavioral activation targets inertia by working from the "outside in" to improve motivation, scheduling activities to allow people to slowly begin increasing their access to mood enhancers. Here's the question for

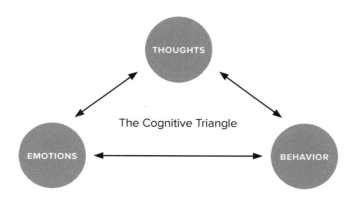

The Cognitive Triangle

a person coping with depression: How much access do you have to rewards if you're isolating yourself? The answer is: probably not much. People who are isolated have less access to things to make them feel better about themselves.

Utilize Reinforcers

Put yourself in a context where you can gain access to rewards, or reinforcers.

Rewards help us feel good and increase our motivation. When we are aware that there could be a potential reward based on our behavior, we are more likely to take action. The concept of scheduling activities that are rewarding is crucial in behavioral activation. When you gradually increase positive activities for yourself, you are rewarded with feeling better and with more motivation. Here are two very simple examples: One scenario brings you further happiness while the other makes you slip deeper into depression.

Example 1: You have a dog you like to take for walks, but today you're feeling depressed. You have two choices: (1) Walk your dog or (2) stay in bed longer. You choose to walk your dog even though you're feeling down. When you go outside, you meet another person who's walking their dog and you notice your mood lift. You feel happier.

Example 2: You have a dog that you normally like to take for walks. You're feeling sad today and decide to sleep in. You don't walk your dog that morning and she has an accident on the carpet. You start blaming yourself for your dog's blunder. You feel more depressed.

Do you have a behavior that causes you to feel more depressed? When you're feeling down it can be hard to change that pattern. Write on the following lines what you're doing that you think is making you feel down.

_____

_____

_____

_____

_____

KAIZEN

Kaizen is the Japanese word for "continual improvement." This concept can be combined with behavioral activation, as it helps us begin to take action by focusing on small steps and then gradually increasing them to bigger ones. For example, Simon likes to run in his rare free time. Sometimes he has automatic thoughts that discourage him from taking that first step out the door. What does he do? He says to himself, "All I have to do is put my running gear on and get outside my front door. If I don't feel motivated to run after I get outside, I can go back in." Simon shares with us that he has never made the choice to turn back after he put on his gear and went outside to exercise. Why? Because he took a small step that resulted in a little boost in motivation, which led to the next step, ultimately leading to a great exercise routine that made him feel good at the end—physically and emotionally.

ACTIVATE BEHAVIOR, CHANGE HOW YOU THINK

When you change your behavior, you will also change the way you think. So another goal of behavioral activation is to change the way you act so that you can create new opportunities to think differently about things. Let's see that in the following example.

Sarah wakes up in the morning and she immediately thinks, "Today's going to be terrible." If she thinks this way, regardless of whether it is accurate, her motivation is going to be low, along with her mood. She may then decide to go back to sleep. If she does that, she's losing the opportunity to be in contact with reinforcers or rewards. Let's say she stays in bed and goes along with the feelings of sadness she's experiencing. Her mood will likely continue to be depressed.

At the end of the day, Sarah hears the phone ring. She may then choose to ignore the phone because her automatic thought is, "No one cares about me, so why should I answer?" She loses another opportunity to be in contact with reinforcers or rewards. How do you think Sarah feels at the end of the day? If you answered, "Even worse," you're likely right.

What could Sarah *do* differently when she has the thought that "today's going to be terrible"?

Take a guess and write on the lines that follow. We'll let you know what Sarah can do differently in a moment.

_____

_____

_____

_____

_____

Behavioral Activation and Depression

Dr. Christopher Martell (one of the creators of behavioral activation) asserts that environmental factors account for depression, and therefore the environment is a more efficient place in which to intervene in order to improve mood. You can have a genetic predisposition to depression (if other members of your family have it), but not everyone with the predisposition becomes depressed, and people with no family history of depression can become depressed. Dr. Martell focuses on behavioral patterns and what is happening in a person's environment to contribute to depression. Maybe the person is isolated and lonely. Perhaps they are having trouble breaking out of a pattern of avoidance that helps them feel better in the short term but is not an effective coping strategy for the long term. That's where behavioral activation comes in. It's a treatment that can help people experiencing depression change what they're doing and in the process begin feeling better about themselves and the life they're living.

PLANNING ACTIVITIES OF PLEASURE AND MASTERY

We all have things we enjoy doing in life, activities that bring us joy and pleasure: things like listening to music, watching a good movie, reading a good book, or eating a good meal. They may not lead to a feeling of accomplishment or mastery, but doing them feels good. We also all have things we may not enjoy doing so much, but we feel a great sense of accomplishment when we've done them: Things like cleaning the bathroom, sorting through mail that has piled up, or doing the laundry. They may not be pleasurable to do, but we feel a sense of mastery once they are done. And some things fit in both categories—they feel good when we do them and we get a sense of accomplishment once they are done. Things like exercise and charitable work might fit here.

When you're feeling depressed, it can be hard to remember what all these things are—and even harder to feel motivated to do them. That's where the weekly activity monitoring and scheduling worksheet can come in handy—it allows you to be more specific about the activities associated with an improvement in mood and in planning when you're willing to try doing these things. Use the following worksheet first to track what your typical day or week looks like in terms of activities and mood levels. Then use it to plan some things you like to do and the times you'd like to do them. It might also help to first generate a big list of the activities you'd think could improve your mood—paying attention to things you used to do, things you currently do (but not as much as you'd like), or things you've never done but predict might help. Also pay attention to all your senses—things you like to smell, taste, touch, see, and hear.

	ACTIVITY (LOCATION, DATE, TIME)
MONDAY	
TUESDAY	
WEDNESDAY	
THURSDAY	
FRIDAY	
SATURDAY	
SUNDAY	

List three activities that bring you pleasure based on the weekly activity monitoring and scheduling worksheet on page 113:

1. _____

2. _____

3. _____

Try doing at least one activity that brings you pleasure each day.

In the table below, rate your level of depression, pleasure, and achievement on a scale of 0-10 before and after each activity.

ACTIVITY (LOCATION, DATE TIME)		DEPRESSION	PLEASURE	ACHIEVEMENT
	Before			
	After			
	Before			
	After			
	Before			
	After			

Feeling Better

Remember how Sarah thought today was going to be awful? Let's see what she could think and do differently to have a better outcome to her day.

Sarah wakes up and she immediately thinks, "Today's going to be terrible." She's already feeling down and she wants to go back to bed. But she reframes her thought and, using the concept of *kaizen*, thinks, "I'm just going to put my feet on the floor and see how I feel." Once she puts her feet down, she realizes that she can stand up. She gets up and notices she's already starting to feel a little bit better now that she's out of bed and activating herself. Then she thinks, "I'm just going to make myself some coffee."

Sarah goes to the kitchen and makes herself a cup of coffee and drinks it slowly. Now she's on a roll! She has another automatic thought: "I don't want to do anything today." But instead of listening to that negative voice, she says to herself, "I'm just going to call Jen to see if she wants to meet up for lunch." She calls her friend and they schedule a time to meet later. Her mood is already beginning to feel better. Why? Because Sarah is (a) activating herself rather than being sedentary, (b) accomplishing small feats, (c) planning a pleasurable activity she can look forward to, and (d) hearing her negative thoughts but not allowing them to prevent

Putting a Stop to Problematic Behavior

Here's an exercise you can try to start changing your behavior. Ask yourself these questions:

1. What do I want to accomplish when I behave this way?

2. How do I feel when I behave this way?

3. Does this behavior impact my relationships? If so, how?

4. What steps can I take to *stop* my behavior?

5. Do I know how to stop it or do I need help from someone else?

her from taking positive steps in the right direction. Now Sarah has numerous chances to be in contact with reinforcers, or rewards.

At the end of the day, because she did not stay in bed, she has a little more energy and motivation, so when she hears the phone ring, she decides to answer it. She may still have the thought that "nobody cares about me," but because she went out and met Jen, she may be more likely to think something less negative. So instead of ignoring the phone, she answers it. It's Jen saying that she had a great time at lunch today. How do you think Sarah feels at the end of the day? If you answered "better" or "happy," you're likely right.

Now that you've thought about the way that your behavior influences your day-to-day life, take a moment to answer the questions about what you can do to stop behavior that is affecting your life negatively. Take out a pen and write on the lines that follow:

_____

_____

_____

_____

Facing Your Fears

Sometimes it can be hard to change your behavior when you're afraid. This is totally valid and understandable. That's where some concepts from exposure therapy can be helpful.

Exposure therapy (which you can do on your own, or, if that's too challenging, under the guidance of a therapist) aims to change your responses to a specific fear. The idea is to gradually and repeatedly confront the thing that frightens you (assuming your fear is excessive and/or unreasonable, relative to how other people would respond to the same trigger), staying in contact with it long enough each time in order to allow your anxiety to peak and then fall, and long enough to learn something new about the trigger or your fears associated with it (i.e., correct inaccurate thoughts). There is a great deal of research suggesting that exposure therapy is very effective at helping people overcome their fears and learn to control their anxiety.

So let's say you want to activate yourself (e.g., go out and meet a friend for lunch), but you need to take public transportation to get there and you're afraid to take the subway. With exposure therapy, you would set up an "exposure hierarchy," with items that provoke less anxiety at the bottom and items that provoke more anxiety at the top. For example, you might first just think about what it would be like to get on a subway car, then you would might walk to the subway station, then you would walk down the steps, then you would buy a subway pass, then you would take the subway one stop, and so on. By systematically breaking your challenge into small steps and facing each one, starting with the easiest step, you should feel your anxiety decrease and your mood increase as you begin achieving your goal of actually riding the subway (i.e., you should feel a sense of accomplishment). Exposure therapy may sound like a slow process, but people often build momentum with each step and, as they gain confidence by succeeding at the smaller initial steps, begin to take on the bigger steps with greater ease. Exposure therapy has successfully helped many people face their fears and is considered by most experts to be the most important ingredient in successful treatment for anxiety. However, it's important to realize that sometimes your fears and anxiety are too challenging to face on your own (i.e., you may also have an anxiety disorder, along with depression). In these cases, consider seeking a therapist who can guide you in confronting and overcoming your fear.

"Avoiding danger is no safer in the long run than outright exposure. The fearful are caught as often as the bold."

—Helen Keller

TYPES OF EXPOSURE

Everybody faces fears differently. Sometimes it can be difficult to confront our fears, and that's perfectly okay. It can take time to face something you've been afraid of for a long time, especially if you've been doing everything you can to avoid triggers and reminders of it. Still, there are ways to face your fears and overcome them. Start by acknowledging your fears and figuring out which exposure method would work best for you. Consider these:

Imaginal exposure. This type of exposure asks the person to picture or imagine their fear in their mind. Let's say you are afraid of filling up your car at the gas station because you will spill gas on yourself. You imagine yourself at the gas station, filling up the car so that you can work through this fear. You can confront this fear by imagining what you would do if you did accidentally spill gas, such as getting help from an attendant.

In vivo exposure. Instead of imagining the scenario, in this type of exposure, you'll be exposed to your fear in real life. For example, if you're afraid of going on an escalator, you'll go to a mall and look at escalators and eventually you'll face that fear by riding an escalator, repeatedly, until you're no longer afraid of doing it.

Virtual reality exposure. In this sort of exposure therapy, the two types of exposure (imaginal and in vivo) are combined. You're put in a situation that seems real but is actually generated by a computer. For example, if you're afraid of spiders, you will experience a simulation of seeing a spider in real life, but the spider is just a computer-generated facsimile. This is a compromise between using your imagination and seeing your fear directly in front of you.

Interoceptive exposure. A person engaged in this type of exposure therapy is exposed to feeling certain body sensations. In this way, he or she gets a more realistic sense of whether or not these sensations pose danger or a threat. The goal is to confront the body sensations and then recognize dysfunctional thoughts that are connected with the feelings in the body. When the individual is able to confront these sensations, he or she learns that they are not dangerous.

Which exposure type might work best for you? What steps do you think would be involved in exposing yourself to the thing you fear? Write about it here:

_____

_____

_____

_____

_____

_____

DIY Exposure Therapy Exercise

1. Generate a list of the things you think make you anxious—these could be situations, places, sensations, images, thoughts, and even feelings.

2. Give each one a rating from 0 (no anxiety) to 10 (extreme anxiety) based on how you think you would feel if you had to face the trigger.

3. Sort the list from lowest to highest.

4. Pick a lower-rated item (e.g., a 3 out of 10) to tackle first. Too low and you may not benefit from the assignment; too high and it may be too difficult to complete.

5. Write down, ahead of time, what you fear will happen and how you will know if it does happen.

6. Conduct your exposure assignment. Stay with it long enough to feel your anxiety reach a peak and begin to fall. (You can do this by noting your anxiety level before, during, and especially after the exercise.)

7. Look for evidence for and especially against your predictions. Note what you learned from doing this exercise.

8. Repeat steps 1 through 7 until the idea of facing that item does not provoke any anxiety (or only minimal anxiety).

Write about your experience here:

_____

_____

_____

_____

_____

_____

_____

_____

_____

Change Your Behavior, Change Your Life

Behavioral activation helps get us unstuck by changing the way we act. You are not your thoughts. Thoughts and feelings are malleable through a change in behaviors. You may feel hopeless at the beginning of the day, but if you activate yourself by engaging in activities of pleasure or mastery, you can help yourself through those feelings and find that your mood will be lifted a little more each day. We believe that you have the power to change the way you think and act. Practice the exercises in this chapter and see if they make a difference in your daily mood.

Review

In this chapter, we talked about behavioral activation. Changing your behavior has the power to change your thoughts and feelings, and vice versa. We went over concrete ways to change problematic behaviors so that they stop affecting your quality of life. When you feel depressed, negative thoughts are going to be there—but they don't have to run your life. We also talked about how fear can have an impact on how we behave and what we think. However, we don't have to let fear stop us from changing our behavior. The strong physiological response associated with fear can literally feel paralyzing, stopping us from moving forward in life. We've discussed how to identify your fears and described different exercises that can help you confront your fears. We've learned about what happens in our brains when we are afraid and how our bodies respond as a result. Exposure therapy is a great technique to help you break down what you're afraid of into smaller, more manageable pieces, which will help you gradually and systematically confront your fear and learn that you can overcome it. However, if your fears or anxiety seem overwhelming or you're not sure where to start, it may be a good idea to seek professional help from a therapist familiar with exposure therapy.

Now you have a better sense of how you can fight back against fear and move forward. Once you face your fear, you will begin to feel more confident. And when you encounter other fears, you'll know what to do with them. What has this chapter illuminated for you? Write about it here:

_____

_____

_____

_____

_____

_____

_____

_____

Homework

This week, you can start by filling out the weekly activity sheet for a day or two. Simply monitor your activity, recording three times a day what you did, the sense of pleasure or mastery (on a scale of 0 to 10) that was associated with each activity, and the impact it had on your mood. Do you see any connections or patterns? If so, you can write about them in the space that follows.

Next, while doing your monitoring, you can also begin generating a list of items of pleasure and mastery (or ideally, both) that you can begin to schedule into your week in order to help yourself feel better. Maybe you want to meet up with a friend, go for a run, or walk your dog.

Fill in the worksheet with your goals for this particular week. When starting, remember the concept of *kaizen*. Remind yourself to start by taking one small step to change your behavior and then see what happens to your motivation and mood afterward (not before). When you're having negative thoughts, see if you are able to deal with them by challenging them, noticing them and letting go, and choosing to behave differently than you typically would, despite what they are telling you to do.

Lastly, if you find that fear is stopping you from engaging in an activity you want to focus on, you can challenge the fear using the steps described in this chapter.

_____

_____

_____

_____

_____

_____

_____

_____

_____

STEP 9

Develop Healthy Lifestyle Habits

Now that you have a better idea of how to talk back to your depression and confront what scares you, it's time to talk about developing some healthy lifestyle habits. Depression can affect every area of your life, and the best way to combat feeling depressed is by engaging in habits that make you feel good physically. Once you feel healthier, the symptoms of depression will be easier to manage. Step 9 focuses on exercise, a healthy diet, taking supplements, and getting outside to help you feel less depressed. Some of these things are intuitive, but you may not have considered some of the others. Even if you're familiar with these tips, it's good to be reminded. This chapter breaks down the elements of a healthy lifestyle so you can begin to incorporate some of these ideas into your daily routine.

The Benefits of Exercise

You likely know that exercise makes you feel better in the abstract sense, but there are many specific reasons why exercise works. Quite simply, exercising regularly improves the condition of your body and mind—getting some physical activity has been proven to enhance quality of life and even lengthen one's life span. Anyone can engage in physical activity, regardless of age, weight, or fitness level. Before you attempt any exercise, speak to your doctor to make sure what you're doing is safe for your body. After that, it's just a matter of finding a routine that's healthy for you and within your ability. Not only is exercise good for everyone but it also specifically benefits people who are living with depression. Let's look at some ways regular exercise can help those of us who are depressed.

BOOSTS ENERGY

Regular cardio exercise, such as walking and running, strengthens the cardiovascular system and conditions the heart and lungs, which can improve your energy levels. It brings oxygen to your body and brain and helps the nutrients you take in reach the right places in your body. When you make exercise a regular part of your routine, you'll discover that you feel better and your daily activities seem easier to accomplish. When Sarah gets outside and goes for a walk, she feels refreshed and motivated to tackle the mundane tasks she needs to accomplish. Being a mom, Sarah is constantly moving and taking care of her kids' needs, and she has incorporated their school pickup and drop-off schedule into her exercise routine—by walking the 2.5 miles to their school, twice daily. This is something you can do, too. Think of ways to integrate exercise into your daily routine. It doesn't have to be an intense workout, just something to help you feel good throughout the day.

RELEASES BRAIN CHEMICALS

During exercise, the body releases "feel-good" chemicals called endorphins, which trigger a positive feeling throughout the body. Chemically, endorphins are similar to morphine (without the danger of addiction), which explains the euphoria that some people may feel after a good workout (the "runner's high," for instance). Generally, when your body feels good, your brain does, too. And as you know, feeling good about yourself goes a long way in relieving some of the symptoms of depression. In fact, according to WebMD, one of the psychological benefits of regular physical activity is higher self-esteem.

Even during periods of depression, you can still experience relief when you do something that releases endorphins into your brain. Think about times in your life when you do find yourself feeling pleasure. What activities give you a dose of those happy chemicals? What lifts your mood, even during times when you're feeling down? Consider all of your senses (sight, smell, taste, sound, and touch) when generating your list. Write your answers here:

_____

_____

_____

_____

_____

_____

GETS YOU INTO SOCIAL SETTINGS

Group exercise is a great way to spend time with other people, together sharing the common goal of getting fit. It's not necessarily about being social (though that might happen with time); it's more about just being around other people. When you regularly attend a class that you enjoy—such as Pilates, yoga, martial arts, or kickboxing—you'll inevitably make some acquaintances. Because you're engaged in the same activity, you share a common bond, which makes for an excellent conversation starter: "How'd you like today's class?" "It was intense, but I got through it."

Although you're ultimately taking a group exercise class to get a good workout, after some time of being exposed to the same people, you might receive (or extend) an invitation to go out for a smoothie. But even if you don't hang with a buddy from the gym, just being around a group of people can make you feel less depressed. Being around other human beings is an essential part of fighting against depression and moving toward a healthier lifestyle.

Other Endorphin-Releasing Activities

Eat chocolate. Cocoa and dark chocolate contain a few mood-brightening ingredients, including phenethylamine and theobromine. When you eat chocolate from time to time, these organic compounds give your brain a nice shot of endorphins.

Enjoy your favorite meal. Chocolate isn't the only feel-good food. When you sit down to your favorite meal, whether that's pizza or a kale smoothie, your brain will enjoy a taste of those happy-making endorphins as you eat.

Laugh. Watch a funny show, tell a friend a silly thing that happened at work, or find another way to laugh your butt off. Laughter is a great way to get those endorphins to pay a visit to your brain.

Get it on. Having sex is a fantastic way to tell your brain to send the endorphins out to play. During sex, you even get a dose of a bonus hormone, oxytocin, which gives you a snuggly feeling of warmth inside.

Listen to music. Hearing your favorite song and singing along is another excellent way to get the endorphins flowing. When your brain registers that the music is pumping, endorphins will show up to the party.

DISTRACTS FROM NEGATIVE THINKING

People have often told Sarah they are in their own heads a lot of the time. This rings true for her, too, as she also tends to overthink things. Sarah finds that regular exercise, whether that's walking or going to a tae kwon do class, helps her accept herself and cope better with feelings of depression or anxiety. Depression often hits hardest when we are alone with our thoughts, and one of the best ways to cope with negative self-talk is by getting up and getting out the door. You may not be able to stop the thoughts, but you can redirect your energy to doing something positive.

"True enjoyment comes from activity of the mind and exercise of the body; the two are ever united."

—Wilhelm von Humboldt

Your Exercise Goals

After reading about the various benefits of exercise, it's your turn to think about how exercise helps improve your mood. Take a moment to think about the type of exercise you enjoy. What helps you feel good both in your mind and body? Do you enjoy swimming, walking, running, or aerobics? Maybe there's an exercise you haven't tried but you're interested in doing. In the space that follows, write down what kind of exercise you like to do and how it makes you feel afterward.

_____

_____

_____

_____

_____

_____

A Sample Exercise Routine

If you don't know where to start, here's a suggested exercise routine to work toward. Before you begin this routine, make sure you consult a medical professional to confirm that it's healthy for you and your body. When you go to the gym, ask for guidance from one of the trainers to make sure you are using the equipment and doing your exercises in a safe and beneficial way. If you exercise at home, watch instructional videos on each type of exercise.

CARDIO. This type of exercise is great for your heart. Try walking or running for 20 to 30 minutes, four to five times a week. Pace yourself and do what you can. Start in shorter increments if necessary.

FLEXIBILITY/STRETCHING. In addition to getting your heart rate up, it's important to stretch your muscles. Do slow stretches for 20 to 30 minutes three times a week. One stretch should last 10 to 30 seconds.

STRENGTH. Do a variety of strength-training exercises to work each of your major muscle groups. The goal is generally 8 to 12 repetitions per set. Try strength training twice a week.

EXERCISE	HOW OFTEN	TIME
Cardio	4 to 5 times/week	20 to 30 minutes
Flexibility/Stretching	3 times/week	10 to 30 minutes
Strength	2 times/week	8 to 12 repetitions per set

Healthy Eating

Eating healthy is essential to maintaining good mental health. Diet doesn't cure depression, but it's an important component to maintaining your physical and mental health. When we feed our body the nutrients it needs, our brain gets the message and we're on the right track to feeling better. There's no specific "depression meal plan," but there are foods you *can* eat to help both your mind and body heal. The goal is to consume foods that contain essential vitamins and minerals. In this section, we're going to examine specific foods involved in creating a healthy and varied diet, focusing on foods that improve brain health. Remember, you don't want to overeat if your appetite is increased; however, it is also important to eat even when your appetite is decreased.

SUPERFOOD MOOD BOOSTERS

From green vegetables and blueberries to fish and eggs, some foods are better at maintaining the health of your brain than others due to their brain-healthy nutrient content. A healthy brain can help you ward off the symptoms of depression. Let's take a look at some good choices to keep in your refrigerator:

Bananas. This popular fruit contains tyrosine, an amino acid that can increase the level of the important feel-good neurotransmitter dopamine. Bananas also contain high levels of vitamin B_6, which helps your brain convert tryptophan into the ultimate feel-good brain chemical serotonin.

> Do you experience insomnia as one of your symptoms of depression? If so, try eating a food that contains the "sleepy" chemical tryptophan before bed. Bananas contain small amounts of tryptophan, and you just might discover that if you eat a banana as a snack before bedtime, you have a better night's sleep.

Berries. Blueberries, blackberries, cranberries, and strawberries all contain the flavonoid anthocyanin. Flavonoids are a group of antioxidants, which are known to help protect the brain from cellular damage as well as fight cancer and other major diseases.

Eggs. Oh eggs, how we adore you for your versatility! Eggs contain amino acids, omega-3 fatty acids, vitamins (A, D, and biotin), and that's not all. They are also rich in minerals, such as zinc and magnesium, which are known to combat anxiety. Eggs are an excellent source of B vitamins, particularly B_{12}, which supports a healthy nervous system. Eggs are also high in protein, so they make the body feel fuller after eating them. They have been known to stabilize blood sugar. Overall, eggs are an excellent choice for your mood and brain health.

Green vegetables. Dark leafy greens such as kale and spinach contain significant amounts of vitamins A, C, E, and K, as well as minerals and phytochemicals. Kale, in particular, is rich in folate, which is an essential nutrient that can help with mood regulation. Some research implicates folate deficiency in the development of major depression.

Salmon. Salmon and other fatty fish are rich in omega-3 fatty acids, which help regulate mood. Other foods, like flaxseed and walnuts, also contain omega-3 fatty acids. If you're a vegetarian (or you just don't dig fish and other sources of omega-3s), you can take an omega-3 fatty acid supplement. Sarah is lucky that she likes salmon and so do her kids. Sprinkle a little soy sauce on that bad boy before cooking, and you're good to go.

According to Melissa Brunetti, a nutritionist who studies the connection between diet and mental health, a great breakfast for someone who is managing depression includes eggs and avocado—a meal rich in omega-3s, vitamin D, and other healthy fatty acids. Include a slice of whole-grain toast, and you have a happy meal for your brain.

What's on Your Menu?

Do certain foods make you happy? Are you a salmon lover? Are you into avocados? How's your scrambled-egg game? Take a moment to think about the foods that make you feel good after you eat them. Now think about the foods that don't make you feel so great. In the space that follows, list the foods that lift your mood and the foods that make you feel down. Next time you're in the store, pick up the feel-good foods and leave the downer foods on the shelf.

There are some foods and beverages that temporarily make you feel good but are not great for your body in the long term. Excessive sugar intake or alcohol consumption (although pleasant in the moment) can often result in more depression later.

The Mediterranean Diet

The Mediterranean diet is rich in fresh fruits and vegetables, whole grains, legumes, lean sources of protein, and olive oil. It's been called one of the healthiest diets in the world. Do you want to incorporate a Mediterranean-style flair into your eating habits? Try these few simple tips:

COOK WITH PLANT-BASED OIL. Olive oil is a great source of monounsaturated fats. You can use it for both cooking and baking. There are other plant-based oils, like canola oil, that are also healthy and contain beneficial omega-3 fatty acids.

EAT LEAN PROTEIN. This starts with eliminating (or at least reducing) red meat from your diet. Try turkey, chicken breast, salmon, or beans. Fish is an especially healthy choice because it is rich in omega-3 fatty acids, which, as you now know, help brain health and improve mood.

EAT MANY SERVINGS OF VEGETABLES. Aim for three to eight ½- to 1-cup servings of vegetables a day. Choose a variety of vegetables in various colors so you can gain the health benefits of different antioxidants, vitamins, and minerals.

MAKE FRUIT YOUR TREAT. If you're like Sarah, you often crave sweets after a nice meal. An excellent way to curb your sweet tooth is to substitute that brownie for some fruit. Fruit is a great way to get your daily fiber, vitamin C, and antioxidants. Fiber is so important to our diets, and we don't eat nearly enough of it. It can prevent the chance of developing colon cancer. After dinner, make a big fruit salad and enjoy!

In the following space, come up with a day's meal plan that incorporates the preceding tips. You don't have to get too specific and create an elaborate menu. Simply jot down some ideas for what you will buy at the store and prepare for breakfast, lunch, dinner, and dessert.

_____

_____

_____

_____

_____

_____

Supplements That May Help with Mood

An important component of maintaining good physical and mental health is getting the right amount of vitamins, minerals, and other essential nutrients. While it's best to get all these nutrients from food, it isn't always possible, so in some cases you'll want to take supplements, too. Here's what to look for:

B vitamins. B vitamins help convert the amino acid tryptophan into the feel-good chemical serotonin, thereby affecting mood and other brain functions. Low levels of B_{12}, as well as vitamin B_6 and folate, have been associated with depression. If your diet is low in B vitamins, a supplement may be the way to go.

Fish oil. Fish oil is an excellent source of omega-3 fatty acids, which help our brains function well and improve our moods. We know from experience that taking cod-liver oil helps lift our mood.

Magnesium. You could call magnesium "nature's chill pill." It's an age-old remedy for relief from anxiety and depression. Magnesium helps cellular and bone health and aids chemical reactions throughout the body. A deficiency in magnesium can reportedly lead to higher levels of depression as well as other physical symptoms, such as muscle tension and headaches. A magnesium supplement may help with depressive symptoms.

Vitamin D. Vitamin D is best known for being a bone-healthy vitamin, but a deficiency in this essential nutrient has been implicated in depression. Because it's found in very few foods, our bodies produce most of our vitamin D in response to exposure to the sun. But, as you know, these days we have to be careful about too much sun exposure, so that's where vitamin D supplements are helpful. In fact, vitamin D supplements are commonly used to treat moderate depression. You can find vitamin D supplements at most pharmacies and grocery stores, or you can get higher doses from your doctor.

Have you tried any of these supplements? Which ones have you tried? Did you notice an improvement in how you feel? If you're curious about giving one of these a try, which one? What do you hope to gain from it? Write about it here:

_____

_____

_____

_____

_____

_____

_____

Review

Hopefully, you've taken away some important information about healthy eating habits, important vitamins, minerals, and supplements that may help your mood, and the importance of sticking to an exercise routine. Remember that it's okay to start slow and pace yourself. We hope that you can integrate the foods and supplements we talked about into your diet. Remember that eating healthy is not a cure for depression; however, it's a crucial aspect of maintaining your mental health. You now have the tools to eat well and take care of your body so that you feel less depressed in the long run. What has this chapter illuminated for you? Write about it here:

_____

_____

_____

_____

_____

Homework

This week, keep a record of the food you eat in the space provided. Next to the food you ate, jot down how it made you feel. You'll likely notice that different foods have different effects on your mood.

_____

_____

_____

_____

_____

_____

_____

_____

Monitor your physical activity this week and note which days you exercised, what type of exercises you did, and for how long. Note which exercises made you feel the best about yourself and stick to doing those in the future. You're on your way to a healthier version of you!

_____

_____

_____

_____

_____

_____

_____

_____

Practice Gratitude and Maintain Mindfulness

Step 10 is a powerful complement to all of the steps described thus far. Consciously being grateful for what you have turns your attention away from what you might be lacking. This practice of gratitude can be an uplifting, positive experience. Along the same lines, being mindful gives you an opportunity to be focused on the present moment. When you are able to stay in the present moment, you aren't dwelling on what happened in the past or what might happen in the future. These practices can relieve suffering, uplift your mood, and help you lead a more fulfilling life. Let's look into some ways to integrate mindfulness and gratitude into your daily routine.

Gratitude Practice

Gratitude is the expression of appreciation for what you have (both tangible and intangible things) as well as for what you have experienced. Gratitude practice is the opposite of dwelling on what you don't have. If you are truly thankful for something or someone in your life, you may find yourself feeling happier. With a regular practice of identifying things for which you are grateful (i.e., counting your blessings), you might notice an increased sense of optimism, leading to feelings of empathy and kindness. Perhaps you'll find yourself more appreciative of what other people bring to your life, and you may even find that others are kinder, too.

IDEAS FOR A DAILY PRACTICE

Not sure where to begin? Here are some ways to start actively practicing gratitude. Try these for a while, and they will likely become second nature:

Keep a gratitude journal. A gratitude journal is a blank notebook where you jot down what you are grateful for. You started this process in step 5 when you listed 10 things you were thankful for. Consider designating a notebook or journal for this purpose and begin by writing down one thing you're grateful for each day. You can return to what you've written occasionally to remind yourself of the positive things in your life.

Regularly tell someone why you appreciate them. Who doesn't love to hear that they're awesome? Take a moment from time to time to call a loved one on the phone to share with that person how they bring you happiness. It'll make you feel good, and it will brighten their day as well. Along these same lines, you can also express your gratitude to coworkers, a helpful salesclerk, a top-notch barista, and so on.

Start small. Think of something small that makes you feel good even for a moment, and be grateful for that. For instance, when Sarah is feeling depressed, she motivates herself by thinking of the little things she is grateful for. If she is lying in bed dreading the start of the day, she brings to mind how good she feels when she drinks her first cup of coffee. Being grateful for that experience motivates Sarah to get out from under the blanket and reward herself with that cup of joe.

Find something to look forward to. Happily anticipating an upcoming vacation is an example of looking forward to something, but it doesn't have to be on such a large scale. Maybe you are looking forward to watching your favorite TV show this evening or finding a new book you'll enjoy. Maybe you're getting together with a friend or family member. Maybe you made an appointment for a manicure. Don't have any plans? You can make a plan and have something fun to look forward to— and be grateful for that.

In the space that follows, list 5 to 10 actions you will take in the next few days to practice gratitude. Does that include keeping a gratitude journal? Calling someone on the phone? Taking a walk in nature? It doesn't matter how big or small these actions are; include them on your list. They matter, and so do you—and that's something to be grateful for.

_____

_____

_____

_____

_____

_____

_____

_____

_____

> When we are grateful, our bodies know it! Research shows that when we focus on thoughts of gratitude, the calming part of our nervous system (the parasympathetic nervous system) is activated, reducing our levels of the stress hormone cortisol and increasing our levels of the "happy" hormone oxytocin.

Be Grateful in the Moment

When you're feeling depressed and need a boost to get you through a particularly difficult moment, stretch your gratitude muscle. Here are a few on-the-spot ideas:

- **DO YOU FEEL TIRED AND ACHY?** Identify an area of your body that feels good. Even if it's just the tip of your nose, place all of your attention there. Think about everything that part of the body does for you and say thank you.

- **BRING TO MIND AN ACT OF KINDNESS THAT YOU DID OR SOMEONE DID FOR YOU, REGARDLESS OF ITS SIZE.** Bask in that feeling of kindhearted-ness for a moment, being thankful for the goodness in the world.

- **IDENTIFY AN ACCOMPLISHMENT YOU'RE PROUD OF.** It could be getting out of bed that morning, washing the car, cooking dinner—whatever it is, acknowledge your ability to accomplish the task. Too often we focus on what we're having trouble with. Instead, be grateful for what you *have* done. (As Sarah wrote this chapter, she remembered that she had already written nine chapters of this book. That made her feel great!)

Mindfulness

Mindfulness is the act of being present in the moment without judgment. You are not engaged in thoughts about the past or the future; you are just here now, observing what is, as it is, not as you'd like it to be. You are aware of the thoughts passing through your mind and sensations in your body, but you don't place negative or positive judgments on them or start analyzing them. You notice them and let them go. You are here, breathing, sitting, standing, or lying down. When you are practicing mindfulness, you feel your feelings and think your thoughts and allow them to be what they are without attaching judgment to them.

How do you feel right now in this moment? Write about your feelings here:

_____

_____

_____

_____

_____

_____

_____

What thoughts are you having right now? Write out some of them here:

_____

_____

_____

_____

_____

_____

_____

NONJUDGMENT IS KEY

Whatever you are feeling or thinking in this moment is perfectly fine. Try not to judge what you are thinking or feeling and try not to judge yourself for having these thoughts or feelings. There's no need to feel any shame around your thoughts and feelings. One of the keys to mindfulness is to put your judgment to the side. Your thoughts and feelings are here, so rather than try to make them something they are not, allow them to be what they are. If you don't try to fight them, chances are you'll be in a better place to work through your thoughts and feelings using the techniques you've been learning throughout this workbook. Be grateful for all your effort up to this point, and keep practicing.

Reread the thoughts and feelings you wrote down in the previous exercise. With an attitude of nonjudgment, sit with those words for a minute. Then, set a timer for five minutes. Close your eyes and practice the mindfulness techniques described in the sidebar on page 142. Be aware, breathe, and sense. Thoughts *will* come into your mind as you do this; that's okay. Let them be there. When the timer goes off, open your eyes.

How do you feel right now in this moment? Write about your feelings here:

_____

_____

_____

_____

_____

_____

_____

_____

_____

_____

Quick Mindfulness Techniques

- **BE AWARE.** Observe your thoughts and emotions in this moment.

- **BREATHE.** Draw your attention to your breath.

- **SENSE.** Notice your body and the physical sensations you are feeling *right now*.

What thoughts are you having right now? Write out some of them here:

_____

_____

_____

_____

_____

_____

Now that you have two sets of thoughts, compare them. Is there a notable difference? Simply observe. There's no correct answer.

THE POWER OF MINDFULNESS AND CBT COMBINED

Both CBT and mindfulness help you become more aware of what's going on in your mind, so they work quite well together. Using mindfulness meditation alongside CBT amplifies your ability to reassess and challenge problematic thoughts and gives you options on how to deal with them—from observing and letting go to reassessing and challenging. As you know, negative thoughts are common (especially in depression), but they are no match for these two powerful tools. Whether or not you are having a depressive episode, incorporating CBT and mindfulness practice into your everyday life can help you exponentially.

Take a look at the thoughts you wrote down in the two previous exercises. Choose one negative thought from among them. You're already familiar with how to use a thought record, but this time, you are going to fill out the worksheet at the same time you are practicing being mindful. Now, write down the negative thought in the thought record worksheet below.

Use the mindfulness technique of withholding judgment. Take a moment to sit with this negative thought on the page. Breathe in and out before you do anything with this thought. See the thought as separate from yourself. If any sensations come up in your body, that's okay. Let them arise.

After you've taken a moment to let this thought sit, see if it still feels as powerful. Is it still front and center in your mind, or were you able to detach from it and let it pass by, like a cloud in the sky? If so, congratulations! You're done. No additional work needed. If not, you can repeat the mindfulness technique and observe what happens this time. Alternatively, you can see if any cognitive distortions are present in your thought (see pages 20 to 22 for a refresher) and complete the thought record worksheet to work through this negative thought.

SITUATION:		
EMOTION:		
NEGATIVE AUTOMATIC THOUGHT:	EVIDENCE THAT SUPPORTS THE THOUGHT:	EVIDENCE THAT DOES NOT SUPPORT THE THOUGHT:
ALTERNATIVE THOUGHTS:		
EMOTION:		

From now on, when you experience negative thoughts (or feelings or sensations), you have two choices: (1) Challenge them by filling out the thought record worksheets or (2) mindfully observe them while withholding judgment. Simply experience them as part of this moment. When you integrate gratitude and mindfulness into your life, you'll begin to see the benefits (slowly at first, but they will continue to grow over time). Your thought records will be the perfect way to look back and see how far you've come.

Here's a worksheet to help you track how mindfulness helps with depression.

SITUATION:		
EMOTION:		
NEGATIVE AUTOMATIC THOUGHT:	MINDFULNESS TECHNIQUE USED:	EVIDENCE THAT DOES NOT SUPPORT THE THOUGHT:
ALTERNATIVE THOUGHTS:		
EMOTION:		

MINDFULNESS MEDITATION

When Sarah was in high school and struggling with anxiety and severe depression, her mom suggested she try mindfulness meditation. Sarah's mom introduced her to a guided meditation by scientist, writer, and meditation teacher Jon Kabat-Zinn, Ph.D. Dr. Kabat-Zinn developed the Mindfulness-Based Stress Reduction program at the University of Massachusetts Medical Center and founded the Center for Mindfulness in Medicine, Health Care, and Society. Dr. Kabat-Zinn's recorded meditations were life changing for Sarah. She was able to sit with her feelings, observe her thoughts in the moment, and feel more relaxed than she did when she started the meditation.

We highly recommend trying mindfulness meditation in either a guided form or by yourself. Many books and recordings are available that will show you how to practice this form of meditation. We've included a sample mindfulness meditation you can do right now (or anytime you'd like):

"Meditation is the only intentional, systematic human activity which at bottom is about not trying to improve yourself or get anywhere else, but simply to realize where you already are."

—Jon Kabat-Zinn

Set aside 30 minutes when you can be by yourself and uninterrupted. (Put that phone away!) Do this in a space where you feel warm and safe. Dress in loose, comfortable clothing that does not constrict your body in any way. Are you ready? Follow these 10 steps:

1. **Find a comfortable position.** You can lie on a mat or on your bed—wherever you feel the most at ease. Close your eyes and take one deep breath in through your nose. Hold it for five seconds. Then release the breath completely.

2. **Take a moment to pay attention to the fact that you are breathing.** This is a beautiful gift. Breathe in slowly through your nose and exhale slowly through your mouth. Each time you exhale, let your body sink deeper and deeper into the surface beneath you.

3. **Notice your feet.** Are you feeling any sensations in them? Tingling, cold, warmth? If you don't feel anything, that's fine. Let the backs of your heels sink into the surface beneath you.

4. **Notice your legs.** Are you feeling any sensations in them? As you breathe in and out, feel your legs getting heavier and heavier. As you shift your attention away from them, release your legs into a deeper level of relaxation.

5. **Now focus your attention on your stomach.** Feel your diaphragm expand as you inhale and release the air as you exhale. Release your stomach muscles and feel them soften with each exhalation.

Five Benefits of Mindfulness

1. **PROVIDES STRESS RELIEF.** Mindfulness calms the mind and body. If you're feeling anxious, a mindfulness meditation can bring your body and mind into a calmer state.

2. **ENHANCES FOCUS.** Mindfulness improves the ability to focus. The more you practice mindfulness meditation, the greater your focus will become.

3. **SUPPORTS CREATIVITY.** Mindfulness helps us be more aware of the negative thoughts that could prevent creative thinking. With those thoughts out of the way, you can place more focus on creative ideas.

4. **IMPROVES EMOTIONAL INTELLIGENCE (EQ).** EQ is our ability to appropriately recognize and respond to feelings in ourselves and others and use our discernment to guide our behaviors and thoughts. Mindfulness helps us better understand our behaviors and deal more appropriately with complex social interactions.

5. **ENCOURAGES KINDNESS AND COMPASSION.** Forbes.com cited a Harvard study that showed a 50 percent increase in kindness and compassion in people who practice meditation, when compared to their non-meditating counterparts.

6. **Shift your attention to your hands.** Squeeze them into fists on the inhalation and completely release them on the exhalation. Feel them becoming heavier.

7. **Turn your attention to your arms.** Are you feeling any sensations in them? Slightly lift your shoulders up as you inhale, and then release them into a deeper state of relaxation and stillness as you exhale.

"Our minds influence the key activity of the brain, which then influences everything; perception, cognition, thoughts and feelings, personal relationships; they're all a projection of you."

—Deepak Chopra

8. **Now notice your throat.** If there is any tension there, breathe into it and let it soften as you exhale.

9. **Move your focus to your jaw.** As you inhale, notice if there is any tension in that area. As you exhale, let your jaw release and relax. Feel your entire face become soft.

10. **Take a deep breath in and notice your whole body.** How is it feeling in this moment? As you exhale, let your body sink deeper and deeper into the surface beneath you. Feel your entire body release and relax. You are in this moment, entirely supported by your body. You are safe and you are loved. As you inhale, think, "I am safe." As you exhale, think, "I am loved."

How did this body scan make you feel? Write down any thoughts, feelings, or body sensations you had following this mindfulness meditation here:

_____

_____

_____

_____

_____

_____

_____

_____

MINDFUL OBSERVATION

Is meditation challenging for you? Here's another exercise you can try to become more mindful. It's called mindful observation. You can do this in your house, on your commute to work, or while walking down the street. Anywhere you find yourself, you'll be able to practice this technique. Follow these four steps:

1. **Wherever you are, select an object to focus on.** It could be a piece of paper, a blade of grass, or a cloud in the sky. It doesn't matter what the object is. You're using it as a focal point. Now, focus on that object for one minute.

2. **Observe this object in its environment.** Try to relax as you watch what this object does or doesn't do. Maybe it sits still the entire time you're watching it or perhaps it's waving in the wind.

3. **Now, observe the object as if you have never seen it before.** Look at each angle of it. Explore its intricate details. What do you notice about it? Are there patterns or colors? Anything else noteworthy?

4. **Reflect on the object's purpose in the world.** What does it provide?

When your thoughts are racing and you can't focus, this is a great way to reset your brain. Do you feel more focused? Are you thinking more clearly? Did it work for you? How did this exercise make you feel? What object did you select? Is there anything you'd like to share about it? Reflect on these questions here:

_____

_____

_____

_____

_____

When you are practicing mindfulness and meditation, it is perfectly normal for your mind to wander. It's part of being human! When it happens, just return your focus to the present moment—as many times as you need to.

Review

We hope you've had an opportunity to practice gratitude and mindfulness so you can see firsthand how it can help you in your daily life. With the information in this chapter, you have the tools to practice both of these techniques anywhere, anytime. You can turn to them in the moment when you need a quick boost of motivation and incorporate them into your daily life along with your CBT techniques—a powerful combo! You don't need to worry about what happened in the past or what's to come. You are here right now. Be grateful for the amazing fact that you are breathing. What has this chapter illuminated for you? Write about it here:

_____

_____

_____

_____

Homework

If you haven't already started keeping a gratitude journal, try it for just this week. You don't have to go out and purchase a fancy journal. A simple notebook will do. Choose the best time for you to set aside 5 to 10 minutes to write in it each day. Write down at least one thing you are grateful for, or if you want to write more, go ahead! At the end of the week, reflect here on how this practice made you feel:

_____

_____

_____

_____

_____

Making It Work

Sarah has never been particularly good at endings. So, let's not think of this as an ending, but rather as the beginning—the start of a better life. If you take anything away from this book, we hope it's this: You can overcome depression with these 10 steps. You may feel overwhelmed by all that you've learned, but you can refer back to any part of this workbook anytime you need a refresher.

Depressive episodes will happen, but that doesn't mean there's anything "wrong" with you. It's okay to feel frustrated, and it's okay to not know what to do. That's why this workbook is here; to give you doable steps you can take to guide you through dark times, even when you feel like giving up. Depression leads you to believe that there's no way out of these dark feelings, but that's a distortion.

The more you practice CBT, mindfulness, and the other strategies in this workbook, the more you will recognize cognitive distortions for what they are and reframe them so that you feel less depressed. Changing your negative thought patterns is challenging, but it is possible. You *do* have the power. You now have the tools to set goals for yourself, and when you stick to your milestones and hold yourself accountable, you'll be able to complete what you set out to accomplish. If your goal is to feel better, then you know how to make that happen.

Remember that sometimes depression can be sneaky and insidious. Don't be hard on yourself if you realize that you are suddenly in the midst of a depressive episode and you didn't see it coming. That's the thing about depression; it doesn't give you a warning, it just shows up and expects you to house it. You can take the Patient Health Questionnaire on pages 6 to 9 from time to time to figure out where you are on the scale if you begin to notice changes. The most important thing to remember is that you didn't "make yourself depressed." And you're not weak or crazy for feeling depressed. There is a pervasive societal stigma about people who experience depression—that they are "being dramatic" or "choosing to feel depressed." This simply isn't true, and we want you to know you didn't bring this on yourself.

We hope you will enjoy practicing your CBT skills. This is a proven therapeutic model for depression that can help you cope with challenging life experiences. As you move through life, you will inevitably have automatic thoughts. With your CBT skills, however, you can identify the cognitive distortion that is at work and manage your thoughts and feelings by creating a thought record. The thought record is probably the most useful tool in this workbook. After consistently working with thought records, you'll find yourself automatically spotting cognitive distortions in your thinking and restructuring them into more balanced, rational thoughts on the spot. As a result, you're less likely to be stuck in a specific depressive episode and more likely to feel mentally balanced in general. There will also likely be a noticeable change in your overall mood and how you cope with life challenges.

You *can* make this work. There's no need to put off taking action. Even if you don't feel like doing the exercises in this book, don't procrastinate. Do them anyway. We know you want to feel better. You don't have to do anything perfectly.

Procrastination arises when we're afraid to move forward, but there's nothing to fear. There is light at the end of the tunnel. Being afraid is a natural part of life, but letting fear run your life isn't necessary. You have strategies for facing your fears now and you know that you will gain confidence when you confront the things that scare you. When you think you can't do something, you can mindfully observe the thought while choosing to push through the fear and do the thing anyway. In other words, you can choose to keep going, even if your mind is telling you that you can't.

A healthy lifestyle that includes a good diet and regular exercise will enhance your mood and overall quality of life. When you have a healthy body, you are more likely to feel better mentally. You don't need to become a gym rat. Start with a few days of brisk walking and build on your new habit from there. And while you're at it, incorporate mindfulness exercises to give your brain a workout, too. Practicing mindfulness and gratitude can be very helpful aids in coping with depression. When you feel depressed, it can be difficult to stay in the moment or be grateful for this moment in time. Being mindful helps us stay open, attentive, and focused on the here and now. It allows you to practice being aware of your thoughts, feelings, and sensations without judging them. Keeping a gratitude journal is a great way to remind yourself of all the wonderful things you have in life, helping you feel more optimistic and positive. Feeling optimistic and positive can help lead you out of depression.

Remember, there is hope. Hope is what keeps us going. You can feel depressed, but within that darkness, know that there is hope. You might not be able to see how things will work out for you yet, but they will. When you're feeling particularly depressed, remind yourself that there is a solution; you just haven't found it yet. Sometimes the solution isn't obvious, but if you keep going and keep searching for a way to work through the problem, it will eventually make itself known. Remember to seek professional help if the techniques in this book don't do the trick or if your symptoms worsen.

It's our sincere hope that you learned a lot from this workbook. In writing it, Sarah was reminded of the many things that help her when she struggles with depression. When we reviewed all the ways to cope with depression outlined here, we left feeling a true sense of hope. We want to leave you with that same hope. Let's take a moment, close our eyes, take a deep breath in, and as we exhale say, "Thank you."

Thank you for reading this book. Thank you for taking this journey with us. We wish you peace and healing through this period of depression. You are stronger than you know.

RESOURCES

If you feel like you are a danger to yourself, please contact the National Suicide Prevention Lifeline at 1-800-273-8255 or SuicidePreventionLifeline.org. Other national hotlines for suicide prevention are geared specifically to the LGBTQ community. They include the Trevor Project at 1-866-488-7386, and Trans Lifeline at 1-877-565-8860 or TransLifeline.org.

Helpful Websites

Find a therapist through these websites:

www.abct.org/Help/?m=mFindHelp&fa=dFindHelp

www.academyofct.org/search/custom.asp?id=4410

https://therapists.psychologytoday.com/rms

http://psychiatry.weill.cornell.edu/cognitive-behavior-therapy-services

www.beckinstitute.org/get-informed/what-is-cognitive-therapy

www.betterhelp.com

www.mayoclinic.org

www.mindfulnesscds.com

www.psychcentral.com

www.psychologytoday.com

www.stigmafighters.com

www.talkspace.com

www.webmd.com

Books

Achor, Shawn. *Before Happiness: The 5 Hidden Keys to Achieving Success, Spreading Happiness, and Sustaining Positive Change.* New York: Crown Business, 2013.

Beck, Aaron T. *Cognitive Therapy and the Emotional Disorders.* New York: Meridian, 1979.

Bourne, Edmund. *The Anxiety and Phobia Workbook.* 6th ed. Oakland, CA: New Harbinger Publications, 2015.

Burns, David D. *Feeling Good: The New Mood Therapy.* New York: Harper, 2009.

Ellis, Keith. *The Magic Lamp: Goal Setting for People Who Hate Setting Goals.* New York: Three Rivers Press, 1998.

Holiday, Ryan. *The Obstacle Is the Way: The Timeless Art of Turning Trials into Triumph.* New York: Portfolio / Penguin, 2014.

Jeffers, Susan. *Feel the Fear . . . and Do It Anyway.* New York: Fawcett Books, 1987.

Kabat-Zinn, Jon. *Wherever You Go, There You Are: Mindfulness Meditation in Everyday Life.* 10th anniversary ed. New York: Hachette Book Group, 2005.

McKay, Matthew, Jeffrey C. Wood, and Jeffrey Brantley. *The Dialectical Behavior Therapy Skills Workbook: Practical DBT Exercises for Learning Mindfulness, Interpersonal Effectiveness, Emotion Regulation and Distress Tolerance.* Oakland, CA: New Harbinger Pubications, 2007.

Peck, M. Scott. *The Road Less Traveled: A New Psychology of Love, Traditional Values and Spiritual Growth.* 25th anniversary ed. New York: Touchstone, 2003.

Rego, Simon A. *Treatment Plans and Interventions for Obsessive-Compulsive Disorder.* Treatment Plans and Interventions for Evidence-Based Psychotherapy. New York: Guilford Press, 2016.

Ruiz, Don Miguel. *The Four Agreements: A Practical Guide to Personal Freedom.* San Rafael, CA: Amber-Allen Publishing, 1997.

Shanahan, Catherine. *Deep Nutrition: Why Your Genes Need Traditional Food.* New York: Flatiron Books, 2017.

REFERENCES

INTRODUCTION

Depression and Bipolar Support Alliance. "Depression Statistics." Accessed September 16, 2017. http://www.dbsalliance.org/site/PageServer?pagename=education_statistics _depression.

Kessler, R. C. "Epidemiology of Women and Depression." *Journal of Affective Disorders* 74, no. 1 (March 2003): 5–13. https://www.ncbi.nlm.nih.gov/pubmed/12646294.

National Institute of Mental Health. "Major Depression Among Adolescents." Accessed September 16, 2017. https://www.nimh.nih.gov/health/statistics/prevalence /major-depression-among-adolescents.shtml.

National Institute of Mental Health. "Major Depression Among Adults." Accessed September 16, 2017. https://www.nimh.nih.gov/health/statistics/prevalence/major -depression-among-adults.shtml.

Son, Sung E., and Jeffrey T. Kirchner. "Depression in Children and Adolescents." *American Family Physician* 62, no. 10 (November 15, 2000): 2297–2308. http://www.aafp.org/afp /2000/1115/p2297.html.

World Health Organization. "Depression." Last modified February 2017. http://www.who.int /mediacentre/factsheets/fs369/en.

STEP 1: DEFINE DEPRESSION

Aaron T. Beck Psychopathology Research Center. "Mission and History." Accessed August 23, 2017. https://aaronbeckcenter.org/about/mission-and-history.

Beck Institute. "Beck Scales." Accessed October 10, 2017. https://www.beckinstitute.org /get-informed/tools-and-resources/professionals/patient-assessment-tools.

Bressert, Steve. "Depression Symptoms (Major Depressive Disorder)." PsychCentral. Accessed August 23, 2017. https://psychcentral.com/disorders/depression/depression -symptoms-major-depressive-disorder.

Harvard Health Publishing. "What Causes Depression?" Accessed September 5, 2017. https://www.health.harvard.edu/mind-and-mood/what-causes-depression.

International Bipolar Foundation. "About Bipolar Disorder." Accessed August 23, 2017. http://ibpf.org/about-bipolar-disorder.

Ko, Jean Y., Karilynn M. Rockhill, Van T. Tong, Brian Morrow, and Sherry L. Farr. "Trends in Postpartum Depressive Symptoms—27 States, 2004, 2008, and 2012." *Morbidity and Mortality Weekly Report* 66, no. 6 (February 17, 2017): 153–158. doi:http://dx.doi.org/10.15585/mmwr.mm6606a1.

Mayo Clinic Staff. "Adult Attention-Deficit/Hyperactivity Disorder (ADHD)." August 15, 2017. http://www.mayoclinic.org/diseases-conditions/adult-adhd/symptoms-causes/syc-20350878.

Mayo Clinic Staff. "Anxiety." August 16, 2017. http://www.mayoclinic.org/diseases-conditions/anxiety/symptoms-causes/syc-20350961.

Mayo Clinic Staff. "Attention-Deficit/Hyperactivity Disorder (ADHD) in Children." August 16, 2017. http://www.mayoclinic.org/diseases-conditions/adhd/symptoms-causes/syc-20350889.

Mayo Clinic Staff. "Persistent Depressive Disorder (Dysthymia)." August 8, 2017. http://www.mayoclinic.org/diseases-conditions/persistent-depressive-disorder/symptoms-causes/dxc-20166596.

Mayo Clinic Staff. "Postpartum Depression." August 11, 2015. http://www.mayoclinic.org/diseases-conditions/postpartum-depression/basics/causes/con-20029130.

Mayo Clinic Staff. "Seasonal Affective Disorder (SAD)." September 12, 2014. http://www.mayoclinic.org/diseases-conditions/seasonal-affective-disorder/basics/definition/con-20021047.

National Institute of Mental Health. "Bipolar Disorder." Accessed August 23, 2017. https://www.nimh.nih.gov/health/publications/bipolar-disorder/index.shtml.

National Institute of Mental Health. "Panic Disorder: When Fear Overwhelms." Accessed August 23, 2017. https://www.nimh.nih.gov/health/publications/panic-disorder-when-fear-overwhelms/index.shtml.

National Institute of Mental Health. "Postpartum Depression Facts." Accessed August 23, 2017. https://www.nimh.nih.gov/health/publications/postpartum-depression-facts/index.shtml.

National Institute of Mental Health. "Seasonal Affective Disorder." Accessed August 23, 2017. https://www.nimh.nih.gov/health/topics/seasonal-affective-disorder/index.shtml.

Sarkis, Stephanie A. "CBT for ADHD: Interview with Mary Solanto, Ph.D." *Psychology Today*. October 11, 2012. https://www.psychologytoday.com/blog/here-there-and-everywhere/201210/cbt-adhd-interview-mary-solanto-phd.

U.S. Department of Veterans Affairs. "PTSD: National Center for PTSD." Last modified August 13, 2015. https://www.ptsd.va.gov/public/problems/depression-and-trauma.asp.

WebMD. "Depression: Recognizing the Physical Signs." Accessed August 23, 2017. https://www.webmd.com/depression/physical-symptoms.

WebMD. "Types of Depression." Accessed August 23, 2017. https://www.webmd.com/depression/guide/depression-types#2-3.

STEP 2: ENGAGE IN THE THERAPEUTIC PROCESS

Beck Institute. "Cognitive Model." Accessed August 23, 2017. https://www.beckinstitute.org/cognitive-model.

Beck Institute. "History of Cognitive Behavior Therapy." Accessed August 23, 2017. https://www.beckinstitute.org/about-beck/our-history/history-of-cognitive-therapy.

Beck, Judith. "The Basic Principles of Cognitive Behavior Therapy." PsychCentral. December 13, 2011. https://pro.psychcentral.com/the-basic-principles-of-cognitive-behavior-therapy/00659.html.

Brownback, Mason and Associates. "10 Principles of Cognitive Behavioral Therapy (CBT)." Accessed August 23, 2017. http://brownbackmason.com/articles/10-principles-of-cognitive-behavioral-therapy-cbt.

EMDR Institute, Inc. "What is EMDR?" Accessed August 28, 2017. http://www.emdr.com/what-is-emdr.

Grohol, John M. "15 Common Cognitive Distortions." PsychCentral. May 17, 2016. https://psychcentral.com/lib/15-common-cognitive-distortions.

Martin, Ben. "In-Depth: Cognitive Behavioral Therapy." PsychCentral. May 17, 2016. https://psychcentral.com/lib/in-depth-cognitive-behavioral-therapy.

National Alliance on Mental Illness. "Psychotherapy." Accessed August 23, 2017. https://www.nami.org/Learn-More/Treatment/Psychotherapy.

National Health Service. "Cognitive Behavioural Therapy (CBT)." Accessed August 23, 2017. http://www.nhs.uk/conditions/Cognitive-behavioural-therapy/Pages/Introduction.aspx.

National Institute of Mental Health. "Borderline Personality Disorder." Last modified August 2016. https://www.nimh.nih.gov/health/topics/borderline-personality-disorder/index.shtml.

RTI International. "Cognitive Behavioral Therapy Can Be as Effective as Second-Generation Antidepressants to Treat Major Depressive Disorder." ScienceDaily. December 9, 2015. https://www.sciencedaily.com/releases/2015/12/151209144936.htm.

WebMD. "Dialectical Behavioral Therapy." Accessed August 23, 2017. https://www.webmd.com/mental-health/dialectical-behavioral-therapy#1.

STEP 3: IDENTIFYING YOUR PROBLEM AREAS

Greenberg, Melanie. "10 Scientific Reasons You're Feeling Depressed." *Psychology Today*. November 12, 2014. https://www.psychologytoday.com/blog/the-mindful-self-express/201411/10-scientific-reasons-you-re-feeling-depressed.

Jang, Yuri, William E. Haley, Brent J. Small, and James A. Mortimer. "The Role of Mastery and Social Resources in the Associations Between Disability and Depression in Later Life." Gerontologist 42, no. 6 (December 1, 2002): 807–813. doi:https://doi.org/10.1093/geront/42.6.807.

Krull, Erika. "Depression and Letting Go of Negative Thoughts." PsychCentral. May 17, 2016. https://psychcentral.com/lib/depression-and-letting-go-of-negative-thoughts.

Krull, Erika. "Replacing Your Negative Thoughts." PsychCentral. May 17, 2016. https://psychcentral.com/lib/replacing-your-negative-thoughts.

Lin, Carrie Elizabeth. "Putting Your Thoughts on Trial: How to Use CBT Thought Records." International Bipolar Foundation. Accessed August 23, 2017. http://www.ibpf.org/blog/putting-your-thoughts-trial-how-use-cbt-thought-records.

Myers, Wyatt. "Depression: How to Challenge Negative Thinking." Everyday Health. Last modified August 6, 2012. https://www.everydayhealth.com/hs/major-depression/how-to-challenge-negative-thinking-from-depression.

Pressman, Sarah D., Karen A. Matthews, Sheldon Cohen, Lynn M. Martire, Michael Scheier, Andrew Baum, and Richard Schulz. "Association of Enjoyable Leisure Activities with Psychological and Physical Well-Being." *Psychosomatic Medicine* 71, no. 7 (September 2009): 725–732. doi:10.1097/PSY.0b013e3181ad7978.

Rodriguez, Tori. "Negative Emotions Are Key to Well-Being." *Scientific American*. May 1, 2013. https://www.scientificamerican.com/article/negative-emotions-key-well-being.

WebMD. "Symptoms of Depression." Accessed August 23, 2017. https://www.webmd.com /depression/guide/detecting-depression#1.

STEP 4: MAKE A PLAN

Grohol, John M. "What Is Catastrophizing?" PsychCentral. May 17, 2016. https://psychcentral.com/lib/what-is-catastrophizing.

Hall, Karyn. "Overcoming Obstacles." *Psychology Today*. May 12, 2016. https://www.psychologytoday.com/blog/pieces-mind/201605/overcoming-obstacles.

University of Michigan Depression Center. *Goal-Setting Worksheet*. Ann Arbor, MI: University of Michigan Depression Center, 2010. http://www.depressiontoolkit.org /download/Goal-settingWorksheet.pdf.

Vilhauer, Jennice. "4 Steps to Finally Accomplish Those Goals You Keep Setting." *Psychology Today*. June 29, 2017. https://www.psychologytoday.com/blog/living-forward/201706 /4-steps-finally-accomplish-those-goals-you-keep-setting.

STEP 5: UNDERSTAND AND IDENTIFY NEGATIVE THOUGHT PATTERNS

Centre for Clinical Interventions. *Improving Self-Esteem*. Module 8: Developing Balanced Core Beliefs. CCI Health. Accessed August 23, 2017. http://www.cci.health.wa.gov.au/docs /SE_Module%208_July%2005.pdf.

Harteneck, Patricia. "7 Ways to Deal with Negative Thoughts." *Psychology Today*. September 29, 2015. https://www.psychologytoday.com/blog/women-s-mental -health-matters/201509/7-ways-deal-negative-thoughts.

Minden, Joel. "Prove It: Overcome Negative Thinking with Targeted Action." *Psychology Today*. April 3, 2017. https://www.psychologytoday.com/blog/cbt-and-me/201704 /prove-it-overcome-negative-thinking-targeted-action.

Psychology Today. "Internal Family Systems Therapy." Accessed August 23, 2017. https://www.psychologytoday.com/therapy-types/internal-family-systems-therapy.

STEP 6: BREAK NEGATIVE THOUGHT PATTERNS

Anderson, Jennifer. "5 Get-Positive Techniques from Cognitive Behavioral Therapy." Everyday Health. Last modified June 12, 2014. https://www.everydayhealth.com/hs /major-depression-living-well/cognitive-behavioral-therapy-techniques.

Cognitive Therapy Guide. "How to Do a Thought Review." CognitiveTherapyGuide.org. Last modified March 1, 2017. http://www.cognitivetherapyguide.org/thought-review -thought-record.htm.

Fredrickson, Barbara L., Michael A. Cohn, Kimberly A. Coffey, Jolynn Pek, and Sandra M. Finkel. "Open Hearts Build Lives: Positive Emotions, Induced Through Loving-Kindness Meditation, Build Consequential Personal Resources." *Journal of Personality and Social Psychology* 95, no. 5 (November 2008): 1045–1062. doi:10.1037/a0013262.

Fredrickson, Barbara L. "Positive Emotions Broaden and Build." In *Advances in Experimental Social Psychology*, vol. 47, edited by Patricia Devine and Ashby Plant, 1–53. Burlington, MA: Academic Press, 2013.

Jordan, Rob. "Stanford Researchers Find Mental Health Prescription: Nature." Stanford News. June 30, 2015. http://news.stanford.edu/2015/06/30/hiking-mental-health-063015.

Lin, Carrie Elizabeth. "Putting Your Thoughts on Trial: How to Use CBT Thought Records." International Bipolar Foundation. Accessed August 23, 2017. http://www.ibpf.org/blog /putting-your-thoughts-trial-how-use-cbt-thought-records.

Mayo Clinic Staff. "Depression and Anxiety: Exercise Eases Symptoms." September 27, 2017. http://www.mayoclinic.org/diseases-conditions/depression/in-depth/depression-and -exercise/art-20046495.

Mayo Clinic Staff. "Positive Thinking: Stop Negative Self-Talk to Reduce Stress." February 18, 2017. http://www.mayoclinic.org/healthy-lifestyle/stress-management/in-depth /positive-thinking/art-20043950.

RN Central. "100 Positive-Thinking Exercises that Will Make Any Patient Healthier and Happier." October 12, 2009. http://www.rncentral.com/nursing-%20library/careplans /100_positive_thinking_exercises_to_incorporate_into_your_life.

STEP 7: DON'T PROCRASTINATE

Boyes, Alice. "6 Tips for Overcoming Anxiety-Related Procrastination." *Psychology Today*. March 13, 2013. https://www.psychologytoday.com/blog/in-practice/201303/6-tips -overcoming-anxiety-related-procrastination.

Cirillo Company. "The Pomodoro Technique." Accessed August 28, 2017. https://cirillocompany.de/pages/pomodoro-technique.

Develop Good Habits. "155 Ways to Reward Yourself for Completing a Goal or Task." Accessed August 28, 2017. https://www.developgoodhabits.com/reward-yourself.

Ethridge, Maggie May. *Atmospheric Disturbances: Scenes From a Marriage.* Bronx, NY: Shebooks, 2014.

Heshmat, Shahram. "The 5 Most Common Reasons We Procrastinate." *Psychology Today.* June 17, 2016. https://www.psychologytoday.com/blog/science-choice/201606/the-5-most -common-reasons-we-procrastinate.

O'Brien, Ed. "Stop Putting Off Fun for After You Finish All Your Work." *Harvard Business Review.* July 7, 2017. https://hbr.org/2017/07/stop-putting-off-fun-for-after-you-finish -all-your-work.

STEP 8: ACTIVATE YOUR BEHAVIOR AND FACE YOUR FEARS

Clark, William R. "Is Our Tendency to Experience Fear and Anxiety Genetic?" *Scientific American.* Accessed August 28, 2017. https://www.scientificamerican.com/article /is-our-tendency-to-experi.

GoodTherapy.org. "Exposure Therapy." Last modified July 3, 2015. https://www.goodtherapy.org/learn-about-therapy/types/exposure-therapy.

Hyman, Ira. "Controlling My Intrusive Thoughts." *Psychology Today.* October 20, 2014. https://www.psychologytoday.com/blog/mental-mishaps/201410/controlling-my -intrusive-thoughts.

Layton, Julia. "How Fear Works." How Stuff Works. Accessed August 28, 2017. http://science.howstuffworks.com/life/inside-the-mind/emotions/fear.htm.

Mayo Clinic Staff. "Specific Phobias." October 19, 2016. http://www.mayoclinic.org /diseases-conditions/specific-phobias/diagnosis-treatment/drc-20355162.

Psychology Today. "Prolonged Exposure Therapy." Accessed August 28, 2017. https://www.psychologytoday.com/therapy-types/prolonged-exposure-therapy.

Shpancer, Noam. "Overcoming Fear: The Only Way Out Is Through." *Psychology Today.* September 20, 2010. https://www.psychologytoday.com/blog/insight-therapy/201009 /overcoming-fear-the-only-way-out-is-through.

Society for the Psychology of Women. "Mary Cover Jones." Accessed October 26, 2017. http://www.apadivisions.org/division-35/about/heritage/mary-jones-biography.aspx.

STEP 9: DEVELOP HEALTHY LIFESTYLE HABITS

Archer, Dale. "Vitamin D Deficiency and Depression." *Psychology Today*. July 11, 2013. https://www.psychologytoday.com/blog/reading-between-the-headlines/201307/vitamin-d-deficiency-and-depression.

Borchard, Therese. "8 Foods that Boost Your Mood." Everyday Health. Last modified July 12, 2016. https://www.everydayhealth.com/columns/therese-borchard-sanity-break/8-foods-that-boost-your-mood.

Domonell, Kristen. "Why Endorphins (and Exercise) Make You Happy." CNN. January 13, 2016. http://www.cnn.com/2016/01/13/health/endorphins-exercise-cause-happiness/index.html.

Goldhill, Olivia. "The Perfect Breakfast for People with Depression." Quartz. July 17, 2016. https://qz.com/734307/the-perfect-breakfast-for-people-with-depression.

Greger, Michael. "Eating Greens Can Fight the Blues: Common Vegetables Help Your Brain Defend Against Depression." *Daily Mail*. March 1, 2016. http://www.dailymail.co.uk/health/article-3472295/Eating-greens-fight-blues-Common-vegetables-help-brain-defend-against-depression.html.

Mayo Clinic. "What Are Omega-3 Fatty Acids From Fish Oil?" August 4, 2016. http://www.mayoclinic.org/what-are-omega-3-fatty-acids-from-fish-oil/art-20232583.

Mayo Clinic Staff. "Depression and Anxiety: Exercise Eases Symptoms." September 27, 2017. http://www.mayoclinic.org/diseases-conditions/depression/in-depth/depression-and-exercise/art-20046495.

Mayo Clinic Staff. "Exercise: 7 Benefits of Regular Physical Activity." October 13, 2016. http://www.mayoclinic.org/healthy-lifestyle/fitness/in-depth/exercise/art-20048389.

Medina, Lily. "Bananas and Depression." Livestrong.com. Last modified August 14, 2017. https://www.livestrong.com/article/164617-bananas-depression.

Migala, Jessica. "8 Ways to Follow the Mediterranean Diet for Better Health." *Eating Well*. Accessed September 1, 2017. http://www.eatingwell.com/article/16372/8-ways-to-follow-the-mediterranean-diet-for-better-health.

Narins, Elizabeth. "11 Ways to Instantly Boost Your Endorphins." *Cosmopolitan*. August 21, 2014. http://www.cosmopolitan.com/health-fitness/advice/a30333/ways-to-boost-your-endorphins.

Penckofer, Sue, Joanne Kouba, Mary Byrn, and Carol Estwing Ferrans. "Vitamin D and Depression: Where Is All the Sunshine?" *Issues in Mental Health Nursing* 31, vol. 6 (June 2010): 385–393. doi:10.3109/01612840903437657.

Physicians Committee for Responsible Medicine. "How Fiber Helps Protect Against Cancer." Accessed September 1, 2017. http://www.pcrm.org/health/cancer-resources/diet-cancer /nutrition/how-fiber-helps-protect-against-cancer.

Stein, Traci. "Depression Won't Go Away? Folate Might Be the Answer." *Psychology Today*. October 6, 2013. https://www.psychologytoday.com/blog/the-integrationist/201310 /depression-wont-go-away-folate-could-be-the-answer.

WebMD. "Exercise and Depression." Accessed September 1, 2017. https://www.webmd.com /depression/guide/exercise-depression#1.

Wei, Marlynn. "Top 10 Foods for a Better Mood." *Psychology Today*. September 15, 2015. https://www.psychologytoday.com/blog/urban-survival/201509/top-10-foods-better-mood.

Wolff, Carina. "5 Foods That Can Help Depression, Because Nutrition Definitely Can Affect Your Mood." Bustle. October 19, 2015. https://www.bustle.com/articles/117751-5-foods -that-can-help-depression-because-nutrition-definitely-can-affect-your-mood.

Zamora, Dulce. "Fitness 101: The Absolute Beginner's Guide to Exercise." WebMD. Accessed September 1, 2017. https://www.webmd.com/fitness-exercise/features/fitness-beginners -guide#4.

STEP 10: PRACTICE GRATITUDE AND MAINTAIN MINDFULNESS

Bradberry, Travis. "Five Ways Mindfulness Will Launch Your Career." *Forbes*. July 6, 2016. https://www.forbes.com/sites/travisbradberry/2016/07/06/five-ways-mindfulness-will -launch-your-career.

Conlon, Ciara. "40 Simple Ways to Practice Gratitude." Lifehack. Accessed September 1, 2017. http://www.lifehack.org/articles/communication/40-simple-ways-practice-gratitude.html.

Dunn, Lauren. "Be Thankful: Science Says Gratitude Is Good for Your Health." *Today*. May 12, 2017. https://www.today.com/health/be-thankful-science-says-gratitude-good -your-health-t58256.

GoodTherapy.org. "Mindfulness-Based Cognitive Therapy." Last modified July 1, 2016. https://www.goodtherapy.org/learn-about-therapy/types/mindfulness-based -cognitive-therapy.

Guided Mindfulness Meditation Practices with Jon Kabat-Zinn. "About the Author." Accessed September 1, 2017. https://www.mindfulnesscds.com/pages/about-the-author.

Lin, Judy. "Mindfulness Reduces Stress, Promotes Resilience." *UCLA Today*. July 29, 2009. http://newsroom.ucla.edu/stories/using-mindfulness-to-reduce-stress-96966.

Niemiec, Ryan M. "Top 10 Things Most People Don't Know About Mindfulness." *Psychology Today*. June 18, 2013. https://www.psychologytoday.com/blog/what-matters-most/201306/top-10-things-most-people-don-t-know-about-mindfulness.

Pocket Mindfulness. "6 Mindfulness Exercises You Can Try Today." Accessed September 1, 2017. https://www.pocketmindfulness.com/6-mindfulness-exercises-you-can-try-today.

Psychology Today. "Gratitude." Accessed September 1, 2017. https://www.psychologytoday.com/basics/gratitude.

Serani, Deborah. "How Gratitude Combats Depression." *Psychology Today*. November 26, 2012. https://www.psychologytoday.com/blog/two-takes-depression/201211/how-gratitude-combats-depression.

INDEX

ACKNOWLEDGMENTS

Sarah—This book was a journey made possible by the incredible people involved in the process. I am honored to have had the chance to work on it. Thank you to Dr. Simon A. Rego for providing essential clinical expertise and making this workbook a place where people can get the help they need. I am humbled to have worked with the staff at Callisto Media, including editors Nana K. Twumasi and Carol Rosenberg—you both have made this process seamless and allowed me to gain invaluable insight throughout the process. And thanks to Marilyn Kretzer and Elizabeth Castoria for believing I could create a book that will help people in distress. Lastly, thank you to the members of the mental health community (including my colleagues at Stigma Fighters), who have continually supported me and led me to where I am today.

Simon—First and foremost, I want to thank my wife, Adriana, for providing me with the support (and time) I needed to work on this project. This book, however, would not have been completed were it not for the talented and ultra-efficient writing of Sarah Fader. Thank you for sharing your anecdotes, Sarah—they really helped the concepts come to life. Thank you as well to Elizabeth Castoria, Nana K. Twumasi, Nichole Kraft, and the rest of the staff at Callisto Media, first for recognizing the power of cognitive behavioral therapy to be so helpful for disorders such as depression, then for providing me the opportunity to get involved with this project, and finally for helping me see it through in such a timely manner. The steps in this book are largely based on concepts created by luminaries in the field of cognitive behavioral therapy such as Dr. Aaron T. Beck, Dr. Judith S. Beck, and Dr. Christopher R. Martell, all of whom I feel very thankful to call my colleagues and to have corresponded with over the years. Finally, I want to thank all of the depressed patients with whom I have worked over the years for having the courage to seek help and for maintaining the conviction that they can get better. Psychological disorders such as depression are real, common, and highly treatable! Please do not lose sight of that.

ABOUT THE AUTHORS

Dr. Simon A. Rego is chief psychologist, director of psychology training, and director of the CBT Training Program at Montefiore Medical Center, as well as associate professor of psychiatry and behavioral sciences at Albert Einstein College of Medicine in New York. He is board-certified in cognitive behavioral psychology, with close to 20 years of experience in cognitive behavior therapy (CBT) for depression, anxiety, stress, and other psychological disorders. He is a member of the board of directors of the Association for Behavioral and Cognitive Therapies, a former member of the board of directors of the Anxiety and Depression Association of America, and a founding member of the New York City Cognitive Behavioral Therapy Association. He enjoys teaching, training, and supervising interns, residents, and fellows on the application of CBT to various psychological disorders, and working with the media to educate the public about the latest mental health news using a simple, non-sensationalized approach.

Sarah Fader is the CEO and founder of Stigma Fighters, a nonprofit organization that encourages individuals with mental illness to share their personal stories. She has been featured in the *New York Times*, the *Washington Post*, the *Atlantic*, *Quartz*, *Psychology Today*, *Huffington Post*, *HuffPost Live*, and *Good Day New York*. Sarah is a native New Yorker who enjoys naps, talking to strangers, and caring for her two small humans and two average-size cats. Like six million other Americans, Sarah lives with panic disorder. Through Stigma Fighters, Sarah hopes to change the world, one mental health stigma at a time. To learn more, visit SarahFader.com.

CPSIA information can be obtained
at www.ICGtesting.com
Printed in the USA
JSHW040503300921
19096JS00004BA/50